Praise for Kristin McGee

and

CHAIR
YOGA

"Kristin is your #1 cheerleader as you pursue your practice."
—Savannah Guthrie

"Kristin is the best combination of skilled and encouraging.
She's as great with a group class of forty-year-old moms
as she is in a private session."
—Tina Fey

"Kristin has been a vital force in my wife's and my yoga for years."
—Steve Martin

"Kristin's approach to yoga is friendly and accessible.
She is hardworking and sweet and helps fit yoga
into your normal life routine."
—Bethenny Frankel

CHAIR
YOGA

KRISTIN McGEE

CHAIR YOGA

Sit, Stretch, and
Strengthen Your Way to a
Happier, Healthier You

wm

WILLIAM MORROW
An Imprint of HarperCollins*Publishers*

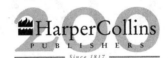

This book contains advice and information relating to health care. It should be used to supplement rather than replace the advice of your doctor or another trained health professional. If you know or suspect you have a health problem, it is recommended that you seek your physician's advice before embarking on any medical program or treatment. All efforts have been made to assure the accuracy of the information contained in this book as of the date of publication. This publisher and the author disclaim liability for any medical outcomes that may occur as a result of applying the methods suggested in this book.

HarperCollins books may be purchased for educational, business, or sales promotional use. For information, please e-mail the Special Markets Department at SPsales@harpercollins.com.

FIRST EDITION

Designed by Diahann Sturge

Boxed abstract lotus symbols © Leone_V/Shutterstock, Inc.

Photography by Chris Fanning (chrisfanning.com)

Library of Congress Cataloging-in-Publication Data has been applied for.

ISBN 978-0-06-248644-8

24 25 26 27 28 LBC 17 16 15 14 13

To my amazing family and to my father,
who never tires of helping his daughter

Contents

Foreword by Sue Hitzmann

Though yoga has been practiced for centuries, there is a need for yoga innovation and modification in our modern age. Much like renovating a classic home, Kristin has reinvented yogic methods to satisfy the needs of a technology-based, seated culture desperate for reacquiring a sense of grounding, movement, and happiness. Her combination of spirit and knowledge has been in the industry from fitness to wellness for many years and my admiration for her perseverance in a field now cluttered with numerous methods of practice is still bountiful. Whether in live classes or on her many DVDs, I always leave her classes feeling uplifted, centered, and more in my body than when I walked in. Much like Kristin, I'm fortunate to have a career that doesn't leave me chair-bound every day, though writing blogs, books, articles, and manuals keeps me at my desk for many hours most days. I know how important it is to have simple, easy techniques to do while at my desk.

Rather than encouraging people to get out of their office to set forth a mindful practice of yoga, Kristin has found simple ways in *Chair Yoga* to bring this beneficial stretching, exercise, and meditative practice to the workspace. I've said in blogs and my own book that sitting is what I consider a "desk sentence" as we are slowly decreasing our vitality from the accumulation of a sitting posture for far too many hours a day. The simplicity of breathing techniques Kristin has set into her book and the many focused exercises and movements she shares may look too easy and thus may be perceived as ineffective. However, knowing these techniques and how she's applied them in *Chair Yoga* can quickly restore balance, focus, and allow a person to regain a sense of well-being in just a few minutes a day. What a great way to prepare for a meeting or interview, or just manage the stress of office life!

Despite the encouragement to have people just get up out of their chairs and move every hour, most people barely get up to go to the bathroom more than once in an afternoon workday. Kristin has thoughtfully compiled movements to keep your face, mind, and body free of tightness that would otherwise cause a workday to feel even more labored.

As technology absorbs our attention both at work and while staring at our phones as we walk down the street, eat lunch, or wait at a stoplight, our need for simple techniques like Kristin's to unwind from our sedentary postures and forward head placement will make this book an added benefit to any lifestyle. Don't let sitting be your desk sentence. It's time to sit up and practice some *Chair Yoga*. You will be better for it. Kristin's mindful and loving ways of enticing people to try something new are captivating. I know as you start to read this book you will soon learn why so many of us in the industry regard her as a key educator in the wellness and fitness community.

Introduction

I'm so happy that you've chosen to move your body throughout your seated day! Chair yoga is the perfect solution for all of us who find ourselves in a chair for extended periods of time. Physical inactivity increases health risks, which is why it's so important to do what you can to add movement throughout your day in order to improve your health. Chair yoga is a practice made up of simple exercises you can do daily that will help strengthen and stretch your body while focusing your mind and helping you tap in to your breath.

Are you living a sedentary life? Do you get out of bed in the morning only to sit down and eat breakfast, sit in a car or on a bus or subway seat on your way to work, sit at a desk all day long, sit on your commute home, sit down for dinner, and then proceed to sit on the couch to watch TV or browse the Internet before you get back into bed?

Does this sound like you? This may be an exaggeration and we all have different jobs. I'm thankful that mine requires me to be on my feet most of the day! But all too many people live sedentary lives, dining, driving, flying, typing, reading, just to name a few activities. It's impossible to escape chairs completely, and we all need to rest our feet at some point in the day. But the balance has tipped. Our early ancestors spent a majority of their time standing and working. As humans, we are designed to move. With our modern-day luxuries and the invention of the television and computers, it is much too easy to spend our days parked on our rear ends.

Sitting Is the New Smoking

The problem with being stuck in a seat all day is finally drawing some attention. Recent studies have shown that sitting in one position for hours can cause major health problems. According to the World Health Organization, physical inactivity is actually the fourth-leading risk factor for death in people around the world.

When we sit all day, we are at risk for developing diabetes, high cholesterol, high blood pressure, postural problems, muscular imbalances, and the list goes on. While we are sitting, our organs aren't required to function at their full capacity; even our lungs don't fully inflate. Plus we lose energy, we develop sciatica, we compress our discs, we lose our abdominal strength, and we age more rapidly. It's rare that someone can sit all day long with perfect posture and awareness.

Many people such as the elderly, those with physical limitations, or individuals who travel for work are forced by circumstances beyond their control to be constantly seated for long periods. Thankfully, there is a solution that can help everyone who finds himself or herself stuck in a seat to feel better, move better, be more productive, and have more energy, awareness, and joy!

What Can We Do About It?

Yoga is the linking of the mind and the body through the breath. Awareness of the breath is key to living a longer, healthier, and fuller life. Yogis use movement, meditation, and breathing exercises to stretch and strengthen their bodies, focus their minds, and improve their well-being. The benefits of yoga are so profound that really everyone should be practicing it in some form.

The very best thing about chair yoga is it can be done *anywhere* and at *any time*! You don't need a mat, you don't have to stand, and you don't need to wear yoga pants–though you can if you want to. Chair yoga is accessible to everyone.

Chair Yoga Can Be Done Anywhere!

Chair yoga is the perfect solution for office workers, commuters, artists, business owners, tired moms, college students, kids, the elderly, the overweight, and couch potatoes and chair spuds everywhere. Chair yoga is the most accessible form of yoga because it can be done in a seat and is easy enough for all levels. It's great for anyone who is deskbound, has limited range of motion, or finds certain traditional yoga postures challenging. Chair yoga can help you become more mindful at work, before you eat a meal, on your travels, or while waiting in a doctor's office. It can be done anywhere and in any type of chair.

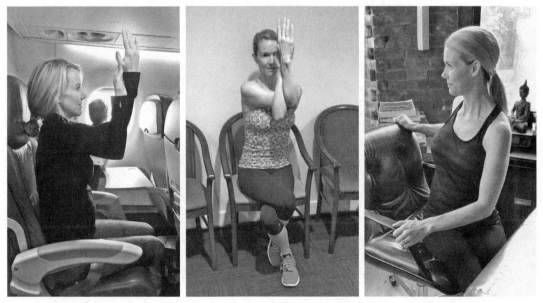

| While on an airplane | Waiting at the doctor's office | While at the office |

Chair Yoga provides a guide to better health with effective, easy-to-follow exercises with step-by-step instructions and photos. Each chapter focuses on stretching and strengthening a different part of the body. It's easy to find five or ten minutes each day to move and breathe and perform these exercises. The benefits to your physical and mental health will be remarkable.

Getting Started

To get started doing chair yoga, all you need is your body, your breath, your willingness, and a chair! If you can start to sneak these exercises into your daily sitting habit, you will find you start to feel better, sleep better, eat better, and have more focus, energy, and stamina. Always keep your breath in mind and let it be your guide for each pose or movement. We'll get to this in the first chapter. You can do any exercise in any order once you connect your mind and breath.

Some days you may find you need a little extra TLC for your wrists, or you need to stand up and get the blood flowing. You are bound to find something in the table of contents that you want to work on, and the best part is that all the exercises can be applied to any kind of seat. We photographed them all in a standard folding chair so that you can better see the anatomical focus and alignment of each pose.

Though you can really pick up this book and start from anywhere, I highly recommend reading chapter one ("Breathe In") first. Once you've mastered the breath, you'll be able to practice the movements of yoga anywhere.

I created this book specifically because so many of us are stuck in chairs all day long. If you find it difficult to fit in movement throughout your day, think of all the places you can do chair yoga, from an airplane to a bus to a doctor's office waiting room to your desk chair to your couch at home. It doesn't matter what you're wearing, what kind of chair you're sitting in, or your environment. The art of yoga is being able to be present anywhere and tap into our vital life force to keep our bodies flexible, strong, and healthy. Let's get started!

1

Breathe In

Without the emphasis on the breath, yoga would be merely stretching and calisthenics. What makes yoga so unique and magical is the breath. Focusing on the breath is one of the easiest habits to develop and implement into your daily routine. Our breath has an instantaneous effect on our overall health and happiness.

Yoga starts with the breath. Breathing practice is referred to as *pranayama,* or "breath control"; we are manipulating the breath to our advantage. *Prana* is Sanskrit for "breath" or "vital energy." On subtle levels, prana represents the energy responsible for our life force. *Ayama* means "control." Therefore, pranayama is "control of the breath." In this chapter you will find various breathing techniques you can use while you practice. These include: *kapalbhati, kumbhaka, sitali, bhastrika, viloma,* and alternate nostril breathing.

The breath is one of our most valuable tools for changing the state of our mind. Have you ever noticed when you're tense or stressed that you hold your breath? Or maybe you take very shallow, rapid breaths all day long because you always feel rushed. Learning to breathe properly can not only help our mental state, but it also makes a huge difference for our physical health and general well-being.

As simple as it sounds, if we aren't breathing, we aren't alive. I remember as a young girl crying uncontrollably, and my dad would say, "Kristin, stop crying and take a deep breath." Once I listened to him, it helped me immediately calm down and change my state of being. Our breath is our life force, and yoga helps us tap into that magical well of energy and life. Every time we pay attention to our breath, we are reminded of how amazing it is to be alive, and thus we are happier, more present, and feel more alert and energized. Tapping into our breath gives us a chance to slow down and get grounded. I know from experience: when I'm not breathing fully, my body feels stiffer, my mind is foggier, and my energy is lower. On the other hand, taking just one deep breath can make a huge change in my demeanor.

How is that so? Taking deep, slow rhythmic inhalations and exhalations through the nose calms the parasympathetic nervous system. Our central nervous system is directly related to our breath. If we aren't breathing properly, the sympathetic nervous system is in a constant state of excitement, setting ourselves up for a state of fight or flight. There are few times when we actually need to activate this feeling (maybe if we are trying to catch a bus, or running from a bear like our ancestors), but mostly we should be calm and centered and oxygenating our bodies fully.

Unfortunately, few of us use our full lung capacity. The good news is that yoga can change all of that.

Tap Into Your Breath

Here is a series of different breathing techniques you can perform in your chair at any time. The key is to take your time to learn how to breathe more fully and exercise your lungs and diaphragm daily. You will notice a huge change in your entire body immediately. By the end of this chapter you will be armed with breathing techniques you can easily incorporate into your daily life.

Ujjayi (Balancing and Calming Breath)

Come into the present moment with this yoga breathing style, which is used when flowing through postures and holding postures.

Helps To: Increase deeper, fuller diaphragmatic breaths, feeding our muscles with extra oxygen

Try This: After a long stint of screen time or whenever you need to relax, focus, or renew your energy

1. Sit comfortably in your chair with your feet flat on the floor. Place on your knees with your palms upward and thumbs and forefingers joined.

2. Inhale a deep breath through your nose, then exhale a silent extended *ha* sound (like Darth Vader) through the mouth. Repeat this two times.

3. Now try creating the silent extended *ha* on both the inhalation and the exhalation but with the mouth closed the entire time. Do this by closing off the back of the throat.

The oceanic sound of the breath is similar to lifting a seashell to your ear. When I first start teaching my students how to breathe, I notice many of them lift their shoulders and breathe only into the upper chest region. *Ujjayi* helps us breathe deeper by bringing the oxygen lower in the body and then filling up the entire chest cavity.

You will use ujjayi breathing during most of the exercises in the chapters ahead and always while you're practicing *asana* (physical postures in yoga). Here are two more ways to practice your ujjayi breathing:

- Try sitting with your feet flat on the floor and your hands on either side of your waist. As you inhale, your hands should move out to the sides as the belly inflates. As you exhale, you'll feel your hands move back in toward each other. Try to exhale every last drop of air out so you have more area to fill up on your next inhale.

- Place one hand on your belly and one on your lower back. As you inhale, imagine the breath going into the hands so you feel your entire body expanding. Before exhaling, place both hands on your shoulders with your palms facing your torso and your fingers wrapped over the tops of the shoulder rims. You should feel your shoulders release.

- Finally place both hands around the small of your lower back and feel the sides of the lower back inflate as you breathe in. This helps you concentrate on filling up the kidney region and forcing your shoulders to stay down.

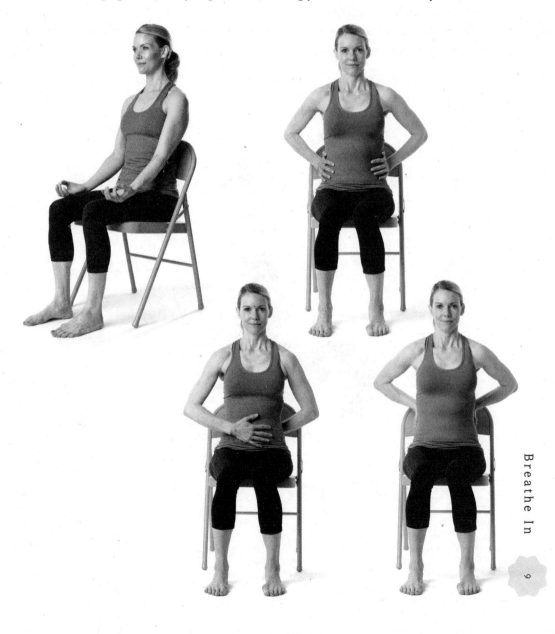

Kapalbhati (Cleansing Breath)

Literally translated as "skull shining," kapalbhati is an awesome way to clean out the cobwebs in the mind and the lungs.

Helps To: Clear the mind, work the core, tone the lower abs, relieve stress, stoke the metabolism, and boost energy

Try This: When you want to wake up, get more energy, or get rid of stale air in the lungs; or before you start a practice or enter a major event

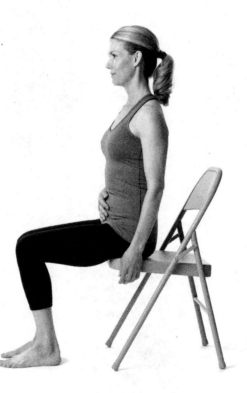

1. Sit tall with your feet firmly planted on the floor.

2. Place your right hand on your belly and relax your left hand on your lap or by your side.

3. Inhale a deep full breath, and then exhale all the air out. Next inhale a partial breath and make short, sharp exhalations out through the nose. You can pump as slow or as fast as you like. The breath is continuous, but the inhalations are very subtle and small. Aim for 80 to 100 pumps or exhalations. You can start smaller with 20 to 30 and build your way up as you develop stamina.

4. At the end of the pumping stop and take a full inhalation and full exhalation.

When you practice kapalbhati you can almost imagine that the air is bouncing off the underside of the brain. Kapalbhati is short, sharp exhalations through the nose with an emphasis only on the out breath.

Kumbhaka (Breath Retention)

Kumbhaka is Sanskrit for "breath retention." It's the practice of holding the breath after an inhalation; it can also be done after all the breath is exhaled out. Kumbhaka is like taking a pause before resuming our breath.

Helps To: Build our lung capacity, give us a moment to feel what it's like to be full or empty, and give us clarity of mind

Try This: When you need a moment of pause, especially after practicing kapalbhati breath

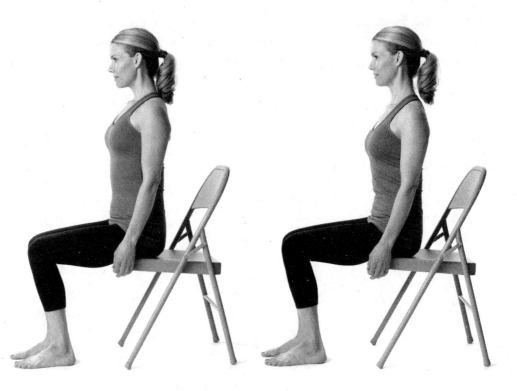

1. Sit tall with your feet hip-width apart and firmly on the floor, and with your hips toward the edge of the chair and your back straight.

2. Take a deep, full breath and imagine the breath circulating in your heart region. Lower your chin toward your chest as you inflate the chest up toward the chin. You can close the eyes for a moment or keep them downcast.

3. Once you can no longer hold the breath in, lift the chin and release all the air out.

4. To add on to this, exhale the air out completely and hold empty for as long as you can before filling up the lungs again.

Alternate Nostril Breathing (Relaxing Breath)

Paying attention to the quality of your breath and following its flow through the nostrils is one of the quickest ways I know of to center yourself. When you are really feeling stressed or frazzled, alternate nostril breathing is your best friend.

Helps To: Boost thinking, calm or reduce agitation, and improve sleep and nasal respiration

Try This: To create a moment of pause, after practicing kapalbhati breath, if you can't fall asleep at night, or to quiet and focus the mind before meditation

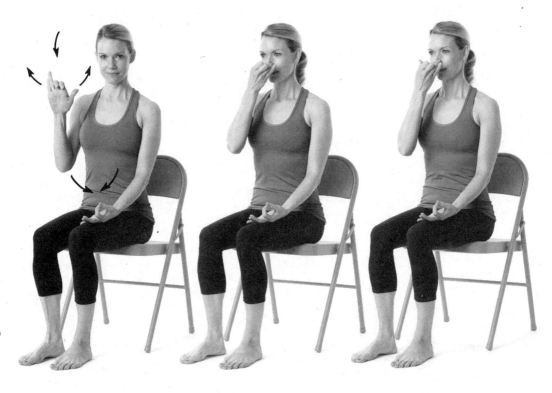

1. Start seated in a nice, tall, comfortable position with your feet on the floor about hip-width apart.

2. With your right hand you'll make Vishnu mudra by bringing the index and middle fingers to the palm and keeping the ring and pinkie finger extended. Your left hand can relax in your lap with the thumb and forefinger joined in *jnana* mudra.

3. Place the thumb on the right nostril and the ring finger on the left nostril and maintain light contact with them the entire time. Gently press the thumb into the right nostril and inhale through the left nostril.

4. Release the thumb from pressing as you close off the left side with the ring finger and exhale out the right side. Inhale through the right, and then press the thumb, gently release the ring finger, and exhale out the left side. Continue going back and forth for at least eight cycles. You can keep your eyes open but slightly downcast or close them.

5. You can also practice this breath without the hand. Imagine the breath passing through each side with the control of the mind.

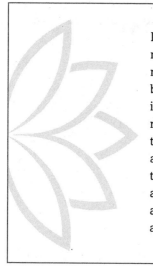

Did you know that over the course of the day, we breathe more predominantly through one nostril for about ninety minutes, then switch to the other nostril? Ancient yogis believed there's a science behind which side we're breathing through and how to use it to be more productive or relax. They thought that breathing in through the left nostril accesses the right "feeling" hemisphere of the brain and helps with relaxation, whereas breathing in through the right side activates the left "thinking" side of the brain and can help energize the mind and body. Consciously alternating between the two sides helps activate and access the entire brain and unites our left and right sides.

As you get more comfortable with alternate nostril breathing, you can start to add retentions and even combine it with kapalbhati breathing. Here are two ways to practice:

- **To Add Retentions:** Inhale through the left side on a slow, steady count (anywhere from 4 to 16) and then close both sides and retain the breath for a certain breath count (can be 4 up to 16, depending on how long you can hold), then exhale out the right side at that same count and keep the breath out for the same count you held in. Continue doing this, lengthening the retention times as you go. For instance, inhale for four seconds, hold for four seconds, exhale for four seconds, and stay empty for four seconds. Maybe eventually you can do eight seconds on each and even build up to sixteen, but only if it's not forced. You want this to be relaxing.

- **For Alternate Nostril Kapalbhati:** Make Vishnu mudra, but this time you'll block off the right nostril and start with short, sharp exhalations out the left side for sixteen counts, then switch and perform sixteen on the right side. Next repeat the exhalations for eight counts on the left side, then eight on the right side, then four, then two, then just back and forth (right, left, right, left, etc.). Finish with either a few cycles of regular alternate nostril breathing or simply breathe clearly and fully through both nostrils and relax.

Bhastrika (Energizing Breath)

Like a traditional bellows that oxygenates a fire and stokes the flames, bhastrika energizes the body and clarifies the mind.

Helps To: Increase prana or life force, build abdominal strength, increase lung capacity, and relieve stress in the brain

Try This: When you're feeling sluggish and need to renew your energy, or to stimulate digestion

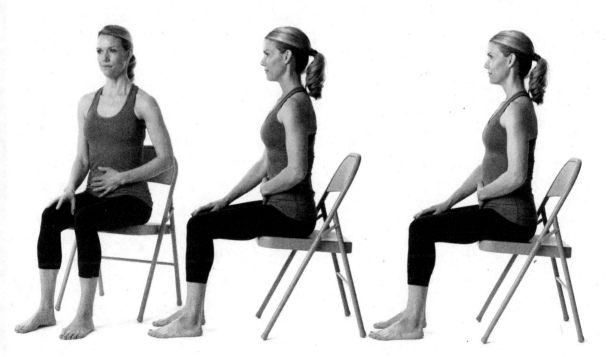

1. Sit tall with your feet hip-width apart and firmly on the floor, and with your hips toward the edge of the chair and your back straight.

2. Inhale a short, forceful inhalation, and then exhale a short, sharp exhalation.

3. Continue in/out, in/out, in/out, over and over again, for at least 30 to 60 seconds.

4. Stop and take a break before repeating again.

5. It can help to place a hand on the belly to feel the abdominals pumping.

Bhastrika is a great way to really energize the entire body and stoke the internal fires. This kind of breath can also be done with movement. Here's how:

- Place your hands on your knees and inhale, sticking your chest out and arching your back. As you exhale, round your spine and pull your chest in. Continue the in/out as you move your spine back and forth for 30 to 60 seconds.

Viloma (Expanding Breath)

Soothing and meditative, viloma breathing pauses on the inhale and exhale, giving us a moment to stop the breath, then resume filling up or letting go.

Helps To: Teach us how to breathe more fully and build our lung capacity
Try This: Toward the end of the day or at the end of a practice

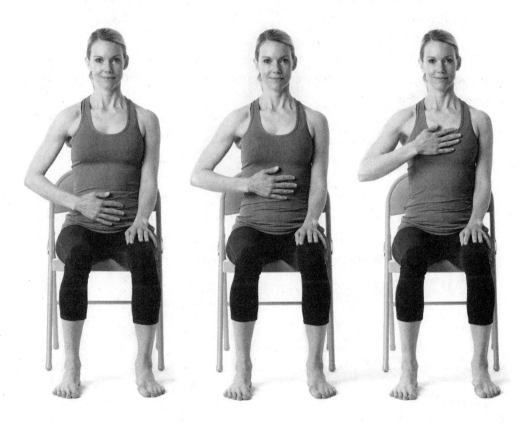

1. Sit tall with your feet hip-width apart and firmly on the floor, and with your hips toward the edge of the chair and your back straight. Inhale and exhale a few normal breaths.

2. Begin inhaling, just to the low belly, then pause; next inhale into your mid-belly and pause; finally inhale all the way up to the tops of your lungs, pause, then exhale all the air out. Repeat this eight times.

3. Now try the pauses on the exhalation. Inhale a full deep breath, then exhale a little and pause, exhale a little more and pause, then exhale all the air out and stay empty for a pause before filling all the way back up. Repeat this eight times.

4. Finally, try the pauses on both the inhalation and the exhalation for a series of eight breaths. You can add as many pauses as you want to, but traditionally this is a three-part breath.

Viloma breathing can also be used as an energizing breath. For the quickest and most natural pick-me-up you have ever experienced (complete with an abundance of energy), try this:

- Inhale at a quicker pace and try breaking the breath up into eight parts, such as inhale, inhale, inhale, inhale, inhale, inhale, inhale, inhale—then release in one long, full exhale. Repeat this 8 to 10 times. Now fill up to the top and let the breath out in eight exhalations with brief pauses in between. Repeat this 8 to 10 times. Finally, try the two together as if you're climbing up a ladder and back down. After 8 to 10 repetitions of the rapid pauses on the inhale and exhale, you will have oxygenated the entire body and brain.

Sithali (Cooling Breath)

Just as animals open their mouths to pant to cool off, sithali breathing helps us cool down. I love this exercise as an alternative to all the breathing exercises that help us warm the body and stimulate energy. There are times when we feel overheated because of our internal or external temperature. In the really hot NYC summer months, I love starting my yoga practice off with a cooling breath.

Helps To: Cool and calm the body

Try This: Any time you're feeling overheated or hotheaded (and need to blow off some steam), or toward the end of the day or at the beginning or end of a yoga practice

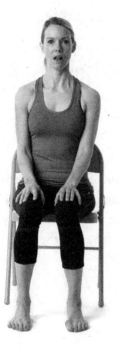

1. Sit tall with your feet hip-width apart and firmly on the floor, and with your hips toward the edge of the chair and your back straight.

2. If you can roll your tongue, do so by curling the sides in toward the center, creating a tube shape; otherwise, just open your mouth and place your tongue on your soft palate.

3. Stick your tongue out between pursed lips or make an O shape with your lips if you can't roll the tongue. Slowly sip in the air. Close the mouth and exhale out the nose. Repeat this 5 to 10 times until you feel a nice, cooling effect.

Sithali is a great breathing tool you can use to cool and calm the body. It's done through a rolled tongue, but not everyone can actually do this—it's a genetic trait. I personally can't! You can also just raise the tongue to the soft palate if rolling your tongue isn't available to you.

2
Warm-ups

By starting off your seated day with these exercises, you will be inspired to move more often throughout your day and to incorporate other stretches and chair poses.

Warming up for any physical activity provides the benefits of injury prevention and enhanced performance. After only 5 to 10 minutes of a warm-up activity, blood flow to the muscles increases by up to 75 percent. In fact, in a study of exercisers where one group warmed up and the other did not, half of the group that warmed up showed improved cardiac effects!

It's traditional in yoga to start with certain warm-ups, often called sun salutations or *vinyasa* (linking breath with movement) flows. Greeting the sun by moving the body with the breath helps put us in a proper mind state to flow more freely and move with more ease. Once you get started, it feels so good it's hard to stop! These exercises are designed to be an easy addition to your day and they really get the blood flowing.

You can think of these flows as moving meditations. So often in life we go about our day aimlessly. When we take the time to link our breath to our movement, our mind and body become aligned and we have a much clearer outlook on our day. We also start to live our life with more purpose and clarity. It's incredible to think that just a few mindful movements can mean so much, but it's true.

Start slowly with any of these exercises and just watch how your day unwinds in a much more calm, focused, energized way. Or try these as you're ending your day before you head home so you have a centered, happy mind and body for your commute and the rest of your evening. I find I will do any of these warm-ups or flows when I'm at the doctor's office, in my airplane seat, commuting on a subway train, or even just hanging out at the end of the day. Give these a try and also feel free to start adding some of your own unique takes on each flow.

Let's Get Started!

You can flow as slowly or as quickly as you like, and your pace may change each time you do the exercises. Listen to your body and your breath and make sure they are linked. Your breathing and your movements should be at the same pace. Make sure you are clear of distractions and your computer and phone are turned off or silenced.

Pelvic Tilts/Circles

Warming up the pelvis and lower abs is one of the first things we often do in our yoga practice. Tapping into the pelvic floor region is great for lifting our energy from the base of our spine upward. I like to think of it as lighting a pilot light at the root of my seat and letting the flame flicker upward. Heating our bodies from the base allows us to access our organic energy and keep the flame going steady all day long.

Works Your: Lower back, pelvic floor muscles, transverse abdominals, and oblique muscles

Try This: When you want to warm up your spine, open up your lower back, loosen up the lower body, engage the pelvic floor muscles, or work the abdominals

1. Sit tall with your feet hip-width apart and firmly on the floor, and with your hips toward the edge of the chair and your back straight.

2. Place your hands on your knees and imagine you have a marble on your belly button and you want it to roll down to your inner thighs; you should feel yourself tip forward onto the fronts of your sitz bones.

3. Pull your belly button to your spine and imagine the marble coming back up the front of your belly to your belly button as you tip your sitz bones underneath you. Try to just isolate the pelvis without tensing the shoulders or arching in the upper back.

4. Continue arching and rounding your lower spine for ten cycles.

5. Next, from the same position, make circles with your pelvis five times in each direction as if you're stirring a pot clockwise and counterclockwise. This movement opens up the lumbar spine and helps us get in touch with our pelvic floor muscles.

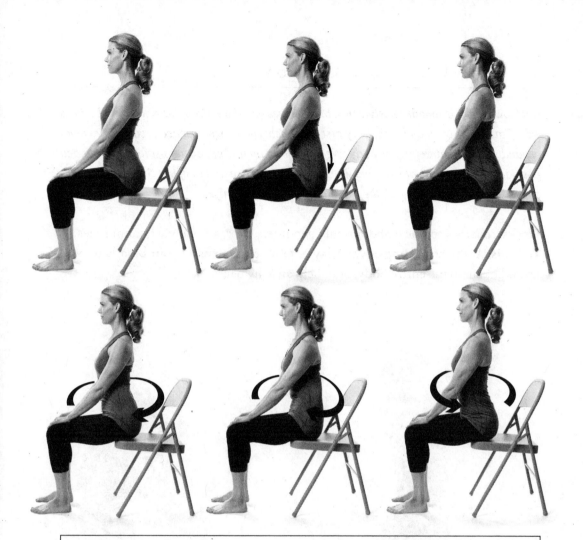

Many Westerners, and especially people who sit in chairs all day, are cut off from their lower half. In Eastern cultures where yoga originated, people squat at the bus stop and use chairs much less often.

They are more in tune with the energy that starts in their seat of power because they charge up from down low as opposed to heating up from the chest upward. We think of our back as starting at our waistband instead of at our tailbone.

When performing this exercise, think about your energy rising from the base of your seat. Do this throughout your day when you feel cut off from your lower half.

Cat/Cow

Cat/cow stretch is similar to pelvic tilts, but it moves into the entire spine and upper body as well. Cat/cow is often one of the very first movements in a yoga practice because it involves expanding and contracting the body. We move from an arched, open position to a rounded position in many of the movements we do in yoga practice and in life. It reminds us to balance everything out and work the front and back body evenly.

Works Your: Spine, back, abdominals, shoulders, hips, and pelvic floor muscles
Try This: At the beginning of your day or practice, to expand your breath, to perk up and open up the entire body, or to help an achy back

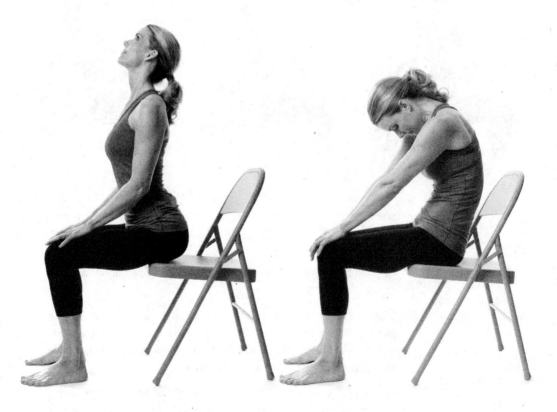

1. Sit tall with your feet hip-width apart and firmly on the floor, and with your hips toward the edge of the chair and your back straight.

2. Place your hands on your knees and inhale, lifting your chest and sticking your hips out behind you. It's as if you're doing the pelvic arch forward but lifting the arch all the way up into your entire back. Lift your gaze, open your chest, and gently squeeze your shoulder blades together.

3. On your exhalation, round your chest, scoop in your belly, and curl under your tailbone as you drop your head toward your sternum (like a Halloween cat).

4. Repeat for a series of ten cycles.

Dancing Cat

I love this exercise, and I named it dancing cat because it really clicks with my students and reminds them to stretch and move the body and limbs as much as possible like a cat does. Cats lie around and stretch all day long!

Works Your: Abdominals, hip flexors, psoas muscles, legs, and pelvic floor muscles
Try This: To give your legs a boost and combat blood clots, work the abdominals and strengthen the core, get your energy going, or stretch the back and spine

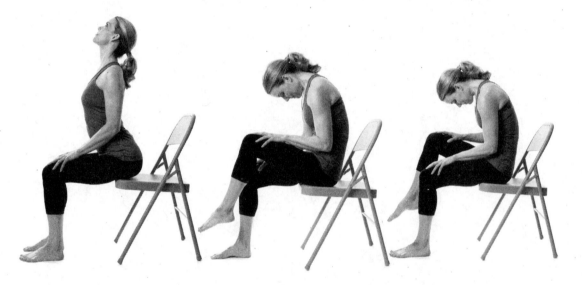

1. Sit at the edge of your seat and perform 1 to 2 rounds of cat/cow.
2. Next inhale to open the back and chest. As you exhale, round the spine and lift your left leg and tuck the knee toward the nose. Repeat with the opposite leg. This is the cat/cow-like movement, but with the knee lift added when you round into the cat shape.
3. Repeat for a series of 8 to 10 repetitions. You may not have the range of motion (or proper garments on) to lift your leg so high at first, but that's okay; just the simple act of feeling the abdominals contract and lifting the foot up off the floor is enough.

Sun Salutations

Sun salutations are a greeting to the sun and a celebration of each and every day. When we take the time to appreciate every day and our opportunity to make the most of our lives, we have a better overall attitude. Performing sun salutations brings the warmth into our body and heats us up. They help give us better circulation, more breath expansion, and increased flexibility.

Sun Salutation Arms • Sun Salutation with Folds

Sun Salutation with Twists • Sun Salutation with Side Bends

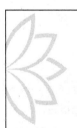

Sun salutations are one of my personal favorites. When we do our sun salutations, it's as if we are opening up to the gifts that the universe has to rain down upon us. We carry so much tension in our shoulders, head, and neck, that it's nice to release the upper body in a flowing way and relieve all the tension so we can sit stress-free.

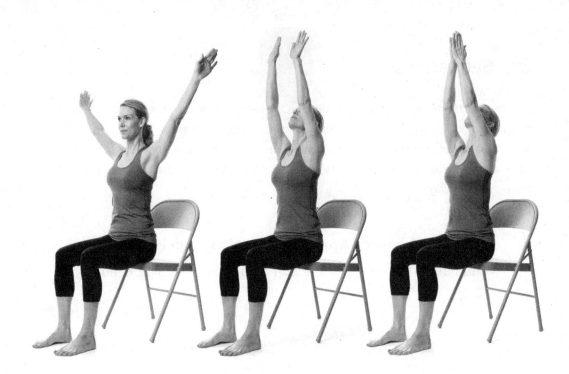

Sun Salutation Arms

Our arms are a direct extension of our heart center region. It can make a world of difference in our mood, energy, compassion, and happiness when we open up our arms and heart and upper body. You can often tell when someone is depressed: his or her shoulders are rounded forward and the chest is caved in. This exercise helps cheer us up and expands our love toward ourselves and others.

Works Your: Arms, shoulders, upper back, and abdominals

Try This: When you need an energy boost, want to rev up your metabolism, feel like you could use some heart opening, or feel a little down or tired

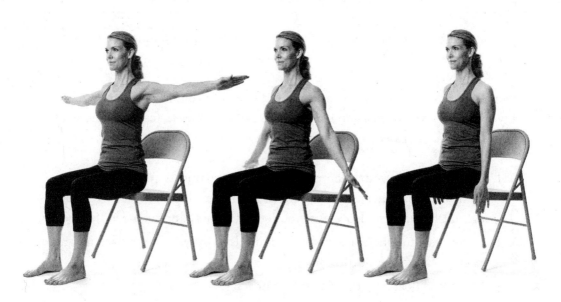

1. Sit tall with your feet hip-width apart and firmly on the floor, and with your hips toward the edge of the chair and your back straight.

2. On an inhalation, lift your arms out to the sides and all the way up overhead (as if making a snow angel). When the arms meet at the top, press the palms together and look up toward them.

3. As you exhale, lower the arms back down until they come to your sides and bring your gaze forward. Take your time as you lift and lower your arms, counting to yourself inhale, inhale, inhale until the arms meet and then exhale, exhale, exhale.

4. Keep your mind in the movement. You will feel muscular energy, but also freedom in the joints and body. This is what yogis refer to as balancing ease with effort. Repeat the sun salutations anywhere from 5 to 15 times.

Sun Salutation with Folds

Now that you've mastered the sun salutation arms, try adding a forward bend to the movement.

Works Your: Spine, back, arms, and abs and stretches your hamstrings and back
Try This: When you need a good hamstring and back release, feel your energy flagging, are feeling stressed, or want to rev up your metabolism

1. Sit at the edge of your chair and start the inhalation as you lift your arms overhead. This time, as you exhale, hinge at your hips and fold over your legs until your torso drops over your lap and your hands come to the floor.

2. As you start to inhale, use your abdominals to lift your torso back up and reach the arms overhead.

3. Exhale and float the arms down to your sides.

4. Repeat this 3 to 5 times, then start to add a small lift of the torso after you fold forward: After you lift the arms up overhead on the inhale and fold forward on the exhale, inhale and look forward from the folded position with the arch out of your lower back. Exhale and fold deeper into your forward bend. Inhale and lift back up with arms overhead; exhale and lower your arms back to your sides. Repeat this combination 3 to 5 times.

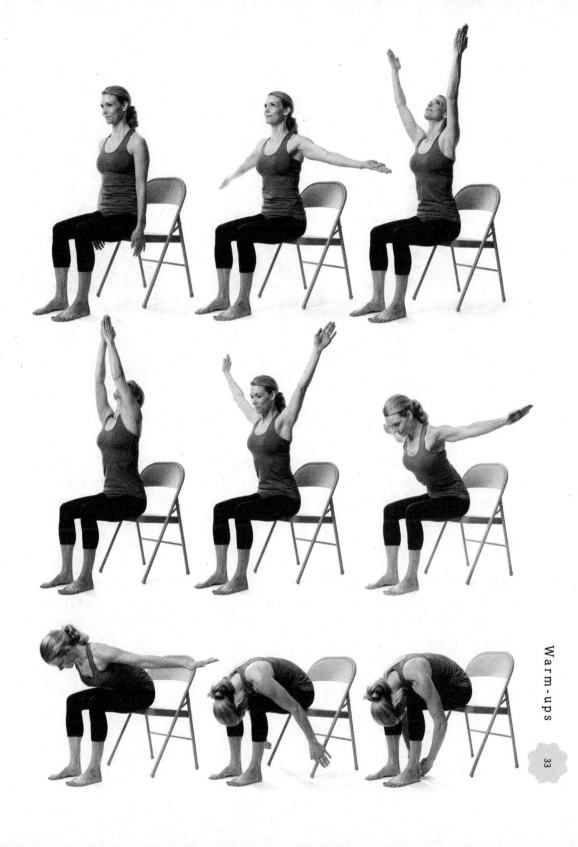

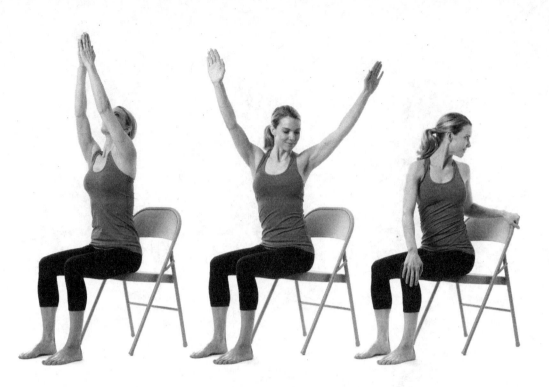

Sun Salutation with Twists

Yoga twists are some of the best things you can do for your spine and core. We use the twisting motion in life so often (getting something out of the backseat of a car; swinging a golf club, tennis racket, or baseball bat; placing things to the side of us; and so on), it's important to twist correctly and keep our bodies safe. Yoga helps us focus on the breath and initiate the twist from the core.

Works Your: Abdominals, spine, lower and upper back, arms, hips, and waist
Try This: When you feel sluggish in your digestion, want to keep your back healthy, feel stuck in your mood or thinking, have a kink in your back or shoulders, or want to wring it all out

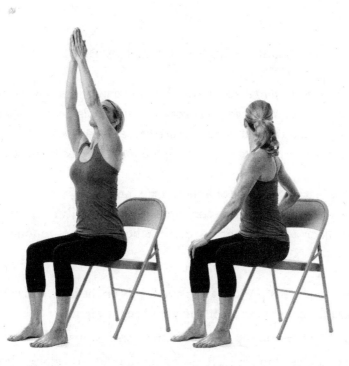

1. Sit tall with your feet hip-width apart and firmly on the floor, and with your hips toward the edge of the chair and your back straight. Inhale, reaching the arms up overhead to press the palms.

2. As you exhale, drop your arms down and around as you twist to your left, bringing the right hand onto the left knee and the left arm behind you to the top of the chair.

3. Inhale back to center with arms up.

4. Exhale and twist to the right.

5. Continue this flow for a series of 8 to 10 cycles. On your last set, stop and hold the twist on each side for 5 to 8 breaths.

> If you feel stuck in any way, twists really help get things moving. Twisting is really good for digestion and detoxification and for seeing things from a new perspective. Twists are also extremely good for the back and waist. You can tone and tighten your oblique muscles and massage the vertebrae of the spine with this flow.

Sun Salutation with Side Bends

When we sit for too long we start to compress our sides and waist and close off our breath. Side bending helps us to sit taller and gain access to deeper, fuller breaths again, and we also boost our energy and clear our minds. Notice how energized you feel after this side-bending flow and also take advantage of all the space you've created in your torso.

Works Your: Abs (particularly the obliques), arms, and back

Try This: When you're feeling a little compressed, need a really great stretch, want to open up the lungs and get more air into the body, or want to tone your love handles

1. Sit tall with your feet hip-width apart and firmly on the floor, and with your hips toward the edge of the chair and your back straight.
2. Inhale and lift your arms up overhead; press your palms at the top.
3. Exhale and side bend to your left, dropping your left arm alongside you as you stretch your right arm overhead. Inhale back up to press palms overhead. Repeat to the other side.
4. Continue flowing from side to side for 8 to 10 reps, and on the final move, hold each side for 5 to 8 breaths.

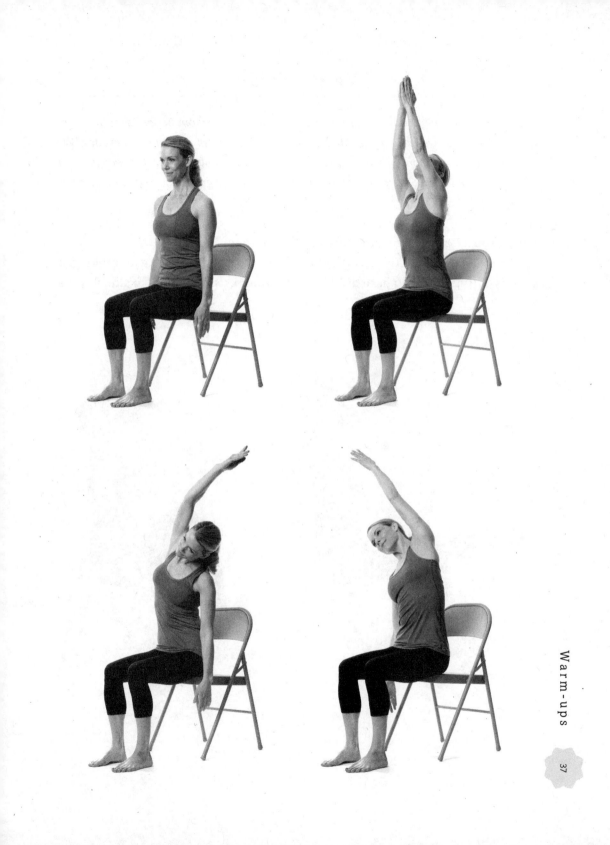

Marching Flow

Get your legs moving to boost your metabolism and get a workout in your seat. So often when we're seated we feel confined and we get bound up in our hips and lower back. We also stay in one position for way too long. The marching flow gets our legs moving and reminds us to mix it up. We concentrate on our large muscle groups in yoga a lot and this flow also gets our lower half warmed up.

Works Your: Core, external rotators, quads, and inner thighs

Try This: If you feel tightness in your lower back or hips, after sitting for prolonged periods of time, or if you have dead butt syndrome or simply want to stretch your legs

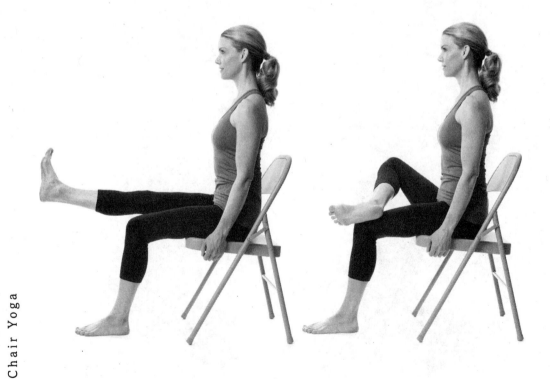

1. Sit tall with your feet hip-width apart and firmly on the floor, and with your hips toward the edge of the chair and your back straight.

2. On an inhalation, extend your right leg straight out in front of you; make sure to engage your quadriceps and lengthen behind the knee.

3. Exhale and bend the knee, opening the right hip as you place the right outer ankle on your left knee (you may need to use your hands to help place the foot and open the leg).

4. Inhale and straighten the leg back forward, then exhale and place the foot on the floor.

5. Repeat the sequence on the left side. Continue this marching exercise 6 to 8 times per leg.

6. On your last repetition, you can keep the knee open and fold forward to stretch out the hip. Hold each side for 5 to 8 breaths.

3

Upper Body

Stopping to give our head, neck, and shoulders a break throughout the day is crucial. The beautiful thing about these stretches and exercises is that they will help your body stay strong while promoting a healthy mind and spirit.

Forward head syndrome, rounded shoulders, computer-related eyestrain—these are all real problems and can result from sitting in a desk seat or chair all day long and using computers, phones, and tablets 24/7. All the exercises in this chapter are incredible for reversing built-up tension.

Our upper bodies hold the weight of the world, and a majority of our tension is often held in our head, neck, and shoulders. It's incredible how often I find myself clenching my jaw or pursing my lips when I'm seated. Many of us wear our shoulders as earrings and end up with major strain in the upper body region. Tight shoulders also affect the wrists and hands and vice versa—if we have tight, weak, or overused wrists and fingers, tension can creep up into the shoulders and neck.

Yoga is truly about longevity and finding a way to maintain our physical body as long as we can. Yoga brings awareness to the ways we misuse our bodies and helps us bring balance back into our life. Sitting for long periods of time at a desk, in a car, on a plane, on a couch, or at a table really isn't ideal for our physical well-being. The exercises in this chapter are an easy way of getting some movement in, particularly in parts of the body that we tend to ignore.

Each one of these stretches can be done independently or in order. Letting go of tension in the head and neck region can make a world of difference in your energy, mood, and even breathing. Our lungs come all the way up to our collarbones, and you won't believe how much more space you can create for full, deep breaths when you free up the head and neck.

Have fun with these moves and open up your upper body in a way that lets you stay strong and flexible, happy and stress-free.

Free Up Tension in Your Head and Neck

We use our brain all day long and it's time we gave it some much-needed TLC. Our head weighs quite a bit, around ten or eleven pounds, and it's a lot of work to support it! Doing these moves feels as good as a massage.

Up/Downs

In this exercise you'll simply lift your head up and down to the rhythm of your breath. This movement frees up the neck and shoulders and allows your body and brain to unwind.

Works Your: Head and neck
Try This: When you want some neck relief, feel tension in your head and neck, or find yourself stuck waiting somewhere

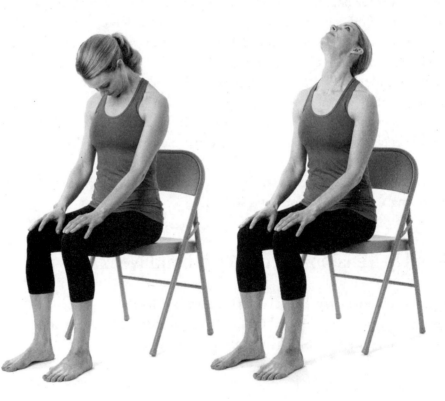

1. Sit tall at the edge of your chair with your feet hip-width apart.

2. Inhale and lift your head up, then exhale and drop your head down. Focus on keeping the torso lifted and isolating the movement in the head and neck.

3. Repeat for a series of ten repetitions.

Side-to-Sides with Neck

Next you'll work on dropping your left ear to your left shoulder, then your right ear to your right shoulder. We carry a lot of tension across the tops of the shoulders into the neck, particularly in the scalene muscles. This exercise helps to release the tension in the neck and it's also good for those of us who carry heavy handbags or briefcases.

Works Your: Head, neck, and upper chest

Try This: After you take off your coat and drop your bag and sit down, when you need some neck release, or when you feel tension across the tops of the shoulders

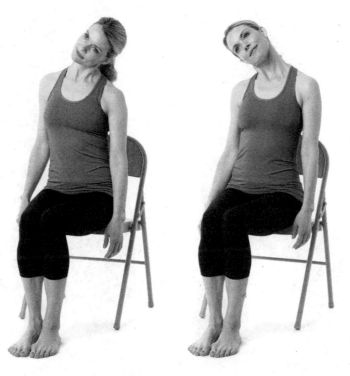

1. Sit tall and on an inhalation let your left ear fall to your left shoulder. Stay for an exhalation, then inhale back up through center and drop the right ear to the right shoulder. Exhale.

2. Inhale and exhale from side to side. Notice how one side can feel much stiffer than the other side. Repeat for a series of ten repetitions.

Right/Lefts

I like this exercise because it helps us gain more mobility in our head and neck region. It also frees up the scalene muscles, which run down the neck to the tops of the shoulders and commonly get tight or really bound up.

Works Your: Head, neck, and upper shoulder regions
Try This: When you want a fresh perspective, need a release across the tops of the shoulders, or feel extra stiff in the head and neck region

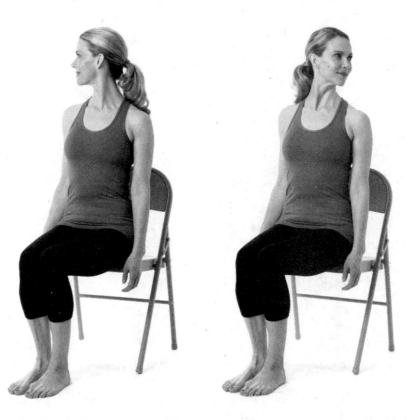

1. Turn your head as far as you can to the right on an inhalation, then turn it as far as you can to the left on an exhalation.

2. Repeat ten times.

Angle Up/Downs

Experimenting with the range of motion in our head and neck region is something we rarely do. Then all of a sudden we find ourselves with a crick in our neck or a weird tightness, and it's uncomfortable and nerve-racking. By keeping our head and neck region limber, and mobile, we decrease our risk of straining or pulling muscles in that region.

Works Your: Head, neck, and shoulders

Try This: When you have unusual stiffness in your neck or want to increase your range of motion

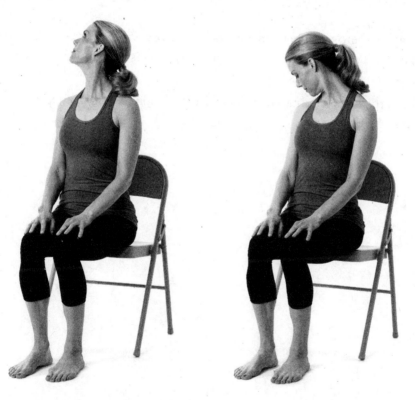

1. Turn your head to your right and lift and lower the head up and down while keeping the head turned.

2. Come back to center and repeat on the left side.

3. Aim for ten repetitions facing right and ten repetitions facing left.

Head Circles

This exercise always reminds me of my old dance stretch warm-ups. Have you ever noticed how free a dancer is in her entire body? Remember the scene from Flashdance *where Jennifer Beals flipped her head around wildly? Finding movement in our upper neck and head region opens us up for more creative thinking.*

Works Your: Head and neck
Try This: When you want to stimulate thought, feel stuck in your work, need a little break, or feel like breaking out your wild child

1. Imagine there's an arrow on your nose and you want to circle it clockwise. Start with small circles, and as your neck warms up you can make them larger.
2. Circle the head ten times in a clockwise direction and then ten times counterclockwise.

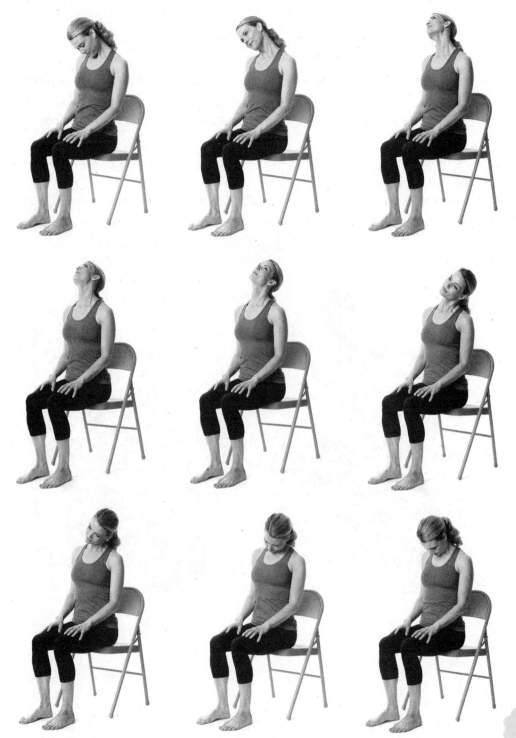

Held Assisted Stretches for Side and Angle

For these next poses, you can stay longer and use your hand to gently prod your head and neck into a deeper stretch. It's lovely when someone else gives us an extra push, but we can also learn to assist ourselves. I find these assisted stretches very meditative and self-soothing.

Works Your: Neck (especially the scalene muscles), upper back (including the trapezius), and shoulders

Try This: When you want some extra TLC, have a headache or neck strain, need some quiet time, or feel a little worn out

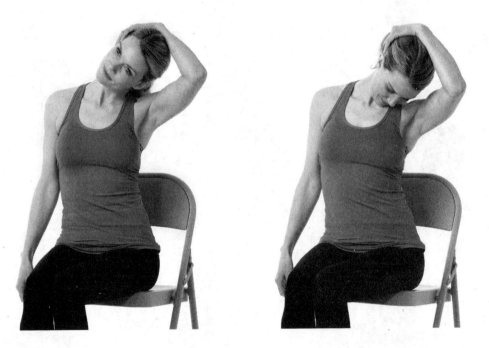

1. Keeping your head looking straight forward, take your left arm overhead to your right ear and drop your left ear toward your left shoulder. Hold the stretch for 8 to 10 breaths.

2. Next turn your chin toward your left armpit while sliding your hand toward the back of your head at the base of your skull. Hold here for 8 to 10 more breaths.

3. Lift your head, drop your arm, and notice the difference in the sides.

4. Repeat on your left side.

Neck Brushing

This exercise stimulates lymphatic flow and helps give us a natural neck-lift. It's also a nice way to release angry thoughts.

Works Your: Neck (including the scalene muscles)
Try This: When you want to stimulate your glands, release any pent-up anger, or smooth out the underside of the neck

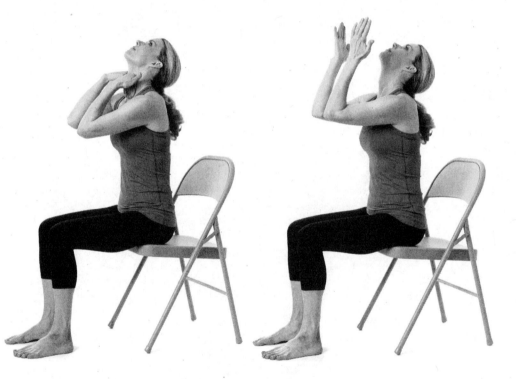

1. Tilt your head up, gazing toward the ceiling, and then use the backs of your hands to brush up the neck, flicking them out at the end of each brush.

2. Try ten brushes or more if it feels good.

Clasped-Hands Head Forward Bow

For major neck relief, you may just want to hang your head forward and use your hands to help let it all go. It's hard to believe how much tension we carry in the neck, and this exercise lets us release it all. It's also a nice way to go inside and turn off all the outer distractions, even if just for a minute.

Works Your: Head, neck, and shoulders

Try This: When you're feeling stressed or overwhelmed, want some major release in the neck, need an entire spine stretch, slept weird, or need a mental or physical break

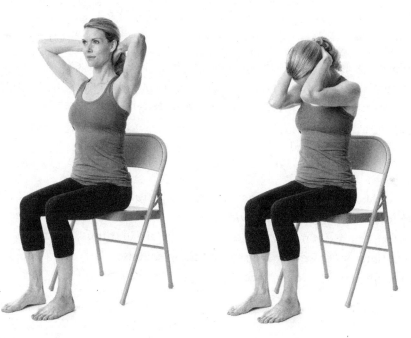

1. Lace your hands behind your head, narrow your elbows forward, and tuck your chin to your chest.

2. Keep your upper body neutral and focus on stretching the upper back and spine. Fold your nose toward your throat region. Hold for at least 5 to 8 breaths.

3. Lift your head up and notice how much relief you feel.

4

Face

How amazing is it to know you have the tools and resources to administer natural Botox to your face? Give yourself a natural face-lift with these exercises as well as reverse and prevent eyestrain and jaw tension.

For all the expensive cleansers, creams, and cosmetics that we use, sometimes we focus too much on improving the skin and ignore the forty-three muscles in our face that we can tone for free! From the circular muscles around our eyes and mouth to the powerful jaw muscles, these exercises can relax the tension and therefore the wrinkles in our face.

I have always suffered from the worst TMJ syndrome. I naturally clench my jaw when I'm concentrating, sleeping, reading, writing, or even performing intense yoga postures. Since I started practicing these yoga face exercises, I've noticed such a difference in my symptoms and pain in my jaw.

I have clients who tell me their eyes constantly hurt from staring at a computer screen all day long. Eyestrain can be alleviated if you stop and do a few simple moves to keep your eyes healthy. Try these whenever your peepers need some relief.

You can go freestyle and just start to move your mouth, jaw, and eyes around to create as many different faces and expressions as you can. It feels so good. Our face is often neglected and yet it's the first thing other people notice about us. Make sure to keep yours relaxed and refreshed by working it out more often.

Since our physicality affects our mentality, even just lifting the corners of your mouth into a smile when you're feeling very down or depressed can get you out of a funk. The second you start pampering yourself with these easy-to-do moves, you'll notice a huge shift in your attitude and health. Plus, in yoga, we never leave out a single body part, from our eyes to our pinkie fingers, bringing awareness to every part of our body. The more we get to know ourselves, the more we appreciate everything our body does for us.

You'll notice that there is no "Works Your" listing for the exercises in this chapter. That's because each exercise works all the muscles of your face, including your eyes, brow, cheeks, jaw, and mouth.

Some people might feel uncomfortable making exaggerated funny faces, but that's exactly what this group of exercises is about. You may want to practice them in front of a mirror. They are perfect for when you're stuck in traffic and need to release stress. These are also easy to do at the end of the day when chilling out on the couch.

Eyes

Up/Downs with Eyes

A simple way to get the eyes warmed up is just looking up and down.

Try This: To start using your eyes in a new way

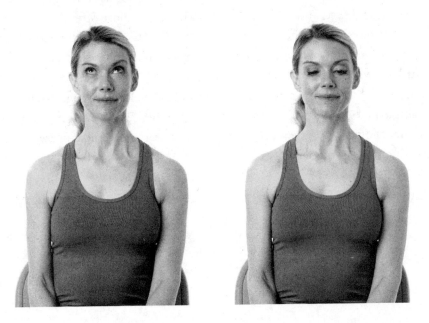

1. Sit in a relaxed position and look up and down with your eyes twelve times. Focus on moving only your eyes.
2. Once finished, relax with your eyes closed for a few seconds.

Side-to-Sides with Eyes

Side-to-sides with the eyes are a little more challenging and make us really focus.

Try This: To stimulate neural activity, exercise the eyes, and create more range of motion in your vision

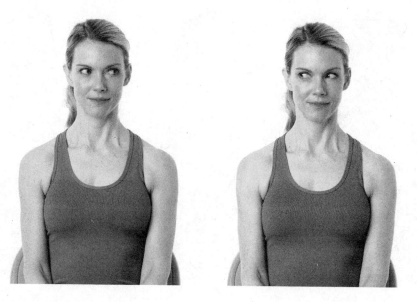

1. Look left and right with the eyes twelve times.
2. Relax with the eyes closed for a few seconds.

Eye Circles

Circling the eyes around is a mind tease! At first it might feel strange (don't overdo it if you feel a little dizzy), but don't worry, over time it will get easier and you'll notice that, like every other part of your body, your eyes, too, need movement in all directions.

Try This: When you need to focus the mind, want a little challenge, or feel like your eyes are getting lazy

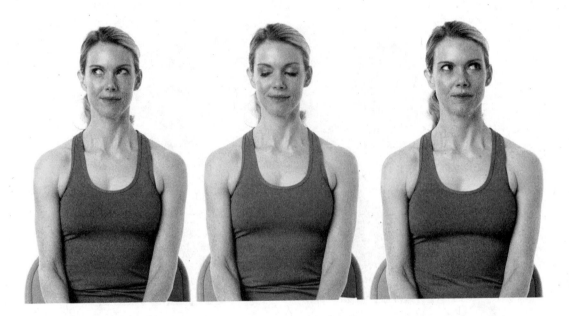

1. Circle the eyes around six times clockwise, then six times counterclockwise.
2. Notice which way is easier and how great this exercise is for focusing the mind.

Close/Opens

Sometimes we just need to shut everything out and go inward. Closing our eyes is one of the easiest ways to do an internal scan. We use our vision for so much input about the world around us. This exercise helps us feel the difference between using our external surroundings and our internal feelings for information.

Try This: When you need a break from staring at a screen, want to experiment with your sense perception, feel your eyes getting tired, or need a little boost

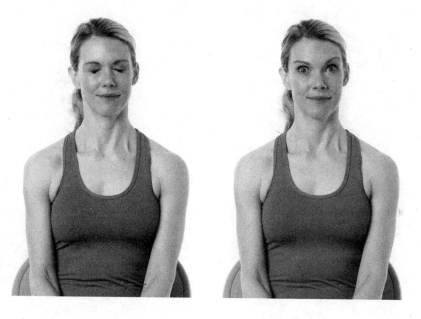

1. Close your eyes for ten seconds.
2. Open your eyes as wide as you can.
3. Repeat for twelve repetitions.

Diagonals

This is the one that always gets me thinking! Eye exercises directly stimulate the brain, and this one in particular works our eyes in directions we aren't used to looking.

Try This: For a little boost, or when you need to balance out your right and left brain, feel you're straining a bit, or are stuck in your seat and need to move something

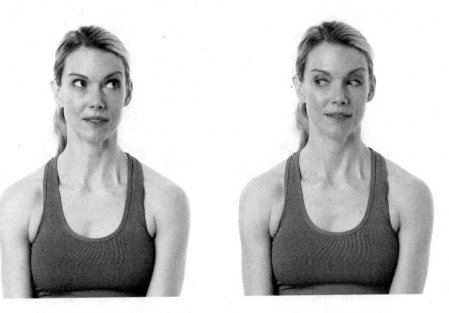

1. Start by looking up to the left at a diagonal, then down to the right at a diagonal. Focus on moving only your eyes. Perform twelve reps of upper left to lower right movements.

2. Next switch and start by looking to the upper right corner and then down to the lower left corner. Repeat upper right to lower left twelve times.

Head Back Downward Gaze

This downward gaze is a nice way to release any tension in your eyes. You will also feel an extra stretch in the front of the neck in a good way.

Try This: For neck and eye relief, a mini vacation for the mind, or a release for the head, neck, and eyes

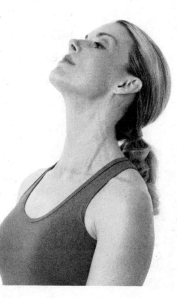

1. Tilt your head back and then gaze down at the tip of the nose.
2. Hold for 5 to 8 breaths.

Mouth

Fishy Face

Sucking in the cheeks isn't just for selfies anymore, plus the practice makes our jowls stronger.

Try This: To warm up your mouth or release mouth tension before speaking in public

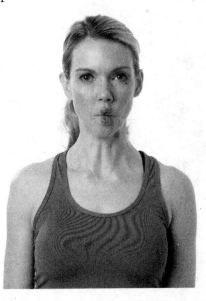

1. Suck in the cheeks and pucker the lips. Hold for three seconds and then release.
2. Repeat ten times.

You may feel silly doing these mouth exercises at first, especially if you're in a workplace environment or surrounded by other people. You may want to start these at home alone, or just find a time when you can get some privacy.

If you start laughing as you do any of these, don't worry! That's always good for the soul no matter what. Eventually you'll come to love how great it feels to work the lips and jaw and mouth.

You'll also appreciate how much younger you look and feel. I do these with my son and we always get a great giggle, and I feel so much looser afterward.

Open Wide

When you really want to release some tension, just open your mouth wide and let it all go! It's unfortunately all too common to go through the day pursing our lips or clenching our jaw. This exercise opens up our mouth and reminds us to release. I think of Macaulay Culkin's expression in Home Alone *when I do this!*

Try This: When you find yourself tensing your jaw, or are feeling overwhelmed and need to release a lot of tension

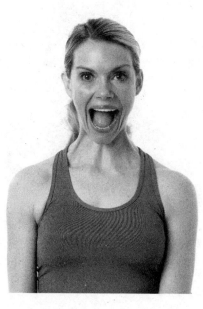

1. Open your mouth as wide as you can.
2. Hold this move for about two seconds and then release. Repeat ten times.

Lower Jaw over Top Teeth

This one is my all-time favorite exercise because I get such relief in my jaw from it. It's a great way to stretch directly under the chin to the front of the neck.

Try This: To stretch out your jaw, to prevent neck wrinkles, or when you need a moment to think

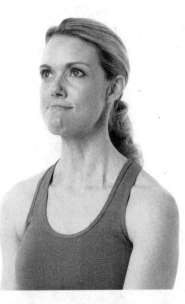

1. Take your lower jaw and lift it over your top teeth. Hold for 15 to 30 seconds. You will stretch the entire underside of the jaw and the neck.

2. Repeat three times.

Side-to-Sides with Lower Jaw

Now that your jaw is a bit looser, you can work on moving it around more and finding its mobility and range of motion. Unless you're an opera singer, stage actor, or trained vocalist, it's not often that you stretch out your facial muscles, mouth, lips, and jaw. Keeping range of motion in our face helps us enunciate better.

Try This: To release jaw tension, to relieve anxiety, or before speaking in public

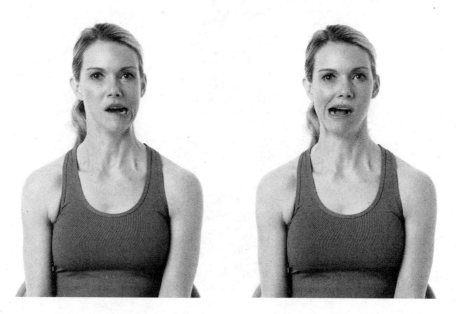

1. Let your lower jaw relax and release from the top jaw, and then try moving it from side to side.

2. Repeat 10 to 15 times.

Gummy Lips

My son often makes this silly face when he's thinking. I started mimicking him and found it freed up my upper lip.

Try This: For more range of motion in your top lip, if you feel stuck in your thinking, or if you are trying to remember something

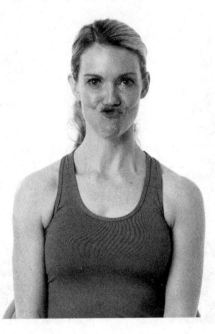

1. Curl your top lip up toward your nose, hold for a few seconds and then release.
2. Repeat ten times.

Wide Smiles

It's true: our expression really does affect our mood. Just by pretending to smile, we feel a lot happier. It's easy to get stuck in a facial posture that's negative or scowl-like. This smile exercise keeps us positive and stretches our face, particularly the lips and mouth.

Try This: To boost your happiness instantly

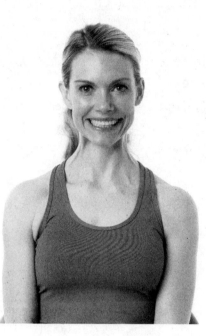

1. Smile as wide as you possibly can, stretching the entire mouth.
2. Hold for a few seconds before relaxing. Repeat ten times.

Lion's Roar

I love to have my students try this pose to break out of their comfort zone. We just aren't used to vocalizing or making crazy faces as adults. If you look at kids, they have so much freedom in their expressions and aren't afraid to make all sorts of silly animal sounds.

Try This: When you really need to let go, have a moment to yourself with no one else around, are with your kids and want to have a fun silly moment, or are stuck in traffic

1. Squeeze your entire face. Really prune it all up—your eyes, forehead, mouth, jaw, everything.

2. Stick your tongue out, open your eyes wide, gazing upward, and *roar* as loud as you can.

3. Repeat as much as you want!

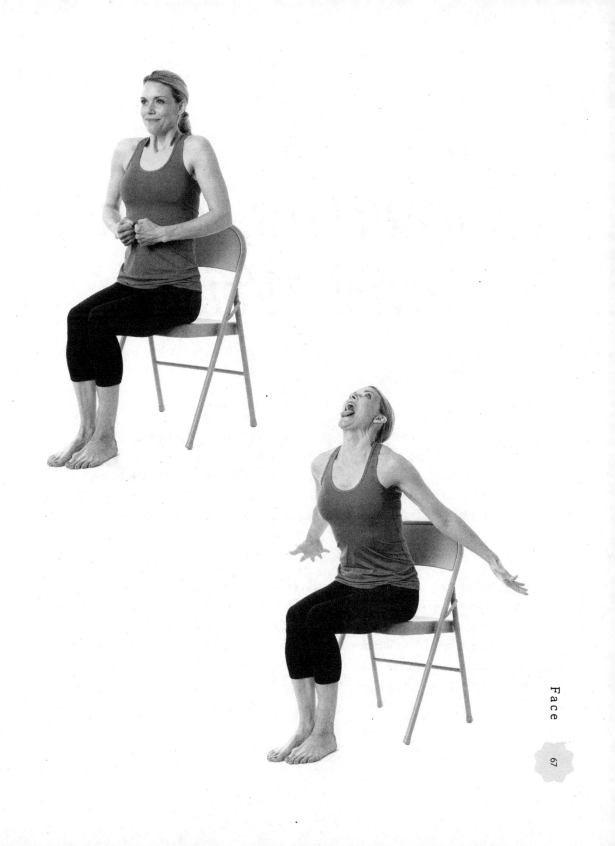

67

5

Shoulders, Arms, and Wrists

There are twenty-nine bones and thirty-four muscles in the hand and fore-arm, so it's important we keep them strong and flexible. The beauty of yoga practice is that it truly leaves nothing out. We work our entire body from head to pinkie finger!

This chapter contains some of my favorite moves to practice regularly. Our arms are an extension of our heart, and the more freedom we can find in our upper body, the easier it is for us to express love to ourselves and to others. I like to think about our arms also as windows. We need to keep them well oiled and be able to open them easily to let in fresh air. When we get all bound up in our upper body, it's so easy to feel stale, frustrated, stressed, and closed off.

Take the time to open the windows, let in a fresh breeze, take deeper and fuller breaths, and let your heart be available in an authentic way. Everyone has a different range of motion, but over time you will be able to make strides with each one of these exercises and get more and more open.

Ever since the invention of computers, portable devices, and smartphones, more people are complaining of pain and discomfort in their hands, fingers, and wrists. When we overstrain our hands, it also affects our arms and sets us up for a whole host of other problems.

It's truly incredible to discover all the ways you can open up your shoulders, arms, and wrists without even getting out of your seat. These stretches will start to become staples for you. Stretching is like flossing your teeth: the more you do it, the easier it gets and the more comfortable it feels. Make it a goal to incorporate some or all of these moves into your daily routine and your heart will feel happier, your body more alive and aligned, your shoulders more relaxed, and your hands and wrists more agile and capable of doing all that needs to be done.

These upper body exercises can be performed pretty much anywhere: at the doctor's office, on an airplane, at your desk, or in the passenger seat of a car. For each movement, try not to overmuscle the pose. It's hard not to tense our shoulders when we work them for some reason. Keep relaxing the tops of the shoulders down away from the ears while you stretch and strengthen the arms, wrists, and shoulders. The very first exercise is one to release the shoulders by overexaggerating how we often have the tops of the shoulders tensed up toward our ears.

This group of exercises stretches, tones, and strengthens the upper extremities. If you feel your arms have gotten a bit flabby or you suffer from certain arm and hand ailments like carpal tunnel, tennis elbow, or texting thumb, these are perfect yoga postures for you.

Shoulder Shrugs

Start out by warming up the shoulders and noticing how much tension you are actually carrying in them. Shoulder shrugs help us to overexaggerate the tension and then fully let it go.

Works Your: Shoulders and lats

Try This: To let go of the stress in your shoulders, sigh it all out, or quickly release the edginess in the shoulders, body, and mind

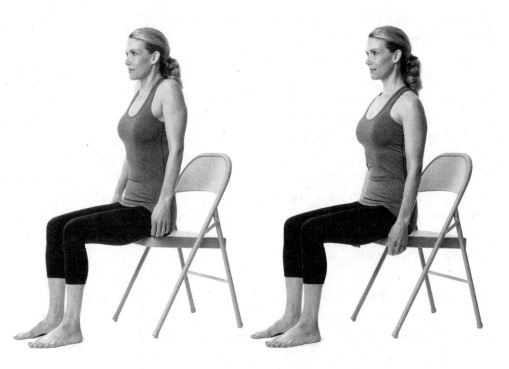

1. Sit tall with your feet hip-width apart and firmly on the floor, and with your hips toward the edge of the chair and your back straight.

2. Inhale and lift the shoulders up toward your ears (as if you were freezing cold); stay tensed for two seconds, then fully release on an exhale. The exhalation can even be sounded like a giant sigh of relief.

3. Repeat 10 to 12 times.

Shoulder Stretch (Arm Across Front)

It's so easy and common to carry tension in our shoulders and neck. This easy shoulder stretch helps to eliminate tightness across the outer arm and the top of the shoulder.

Works Your: Outer shoulder, rear deltoid, and biceps

Try This: When you need a release in the shoulder, head, and neck region; feel stiff in the neck; have had an intense workout; notice your shoulders creeping up to your ears; or want a good prep for eagle arms

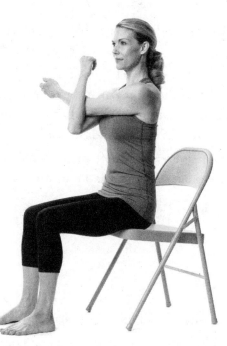

1. Sit tall at the edge of your seat.

2. Take your left arm straight across the front of the body as you use your right arm to pull it in closer to your midline.

3. Keep the top of the shoulder released down away from the ear and hold and breathe for 5 to 8 breaths.

4. Repeat on the right side.

Eagle Arms

Eagle pose is said to be good for focusing the mind and concentrating on your breath. It also opens up our shoulders, upper back, elbows, and wrists. When we perform eagle arms, we are working the tops of the shoulders down away from the ears. It's such a wonderful feeling to find a concentrated level of focus while keeping our shoulders relaxed.

Works Your: Arms, wrists, and shoulders
Try This: When you need some wrist and shoulder relief

1. Sit tall with your feet hip-width apart and firmly on the floor, and with your hips toward the edge of the chair and your back straight. Take your arms out to the sides at shoulder height, palms open to the ceiling.

2. Wrap the left arm under the right arm as high up as you can, then double cross the forearms and try to press the palms together. If you can't touch your palms, press the backs of the hands instead.

3. Work on lifting your elbows while softening your shoulders. Hold for 5 to 8 breaths before releasing the arms and repeating with the opposite arm crossing.

Variations:

1. Once you're in eagle arms position, lift the arms up and down three times.

2. Try circling the arms clockwise three times and counterclockwise three times.

3. Stretch the position to the right and look to the left for five breaths, then take the arms to the left as you look to the right for five breaths.

4. Repeat each variation with the opposite arm crossing.

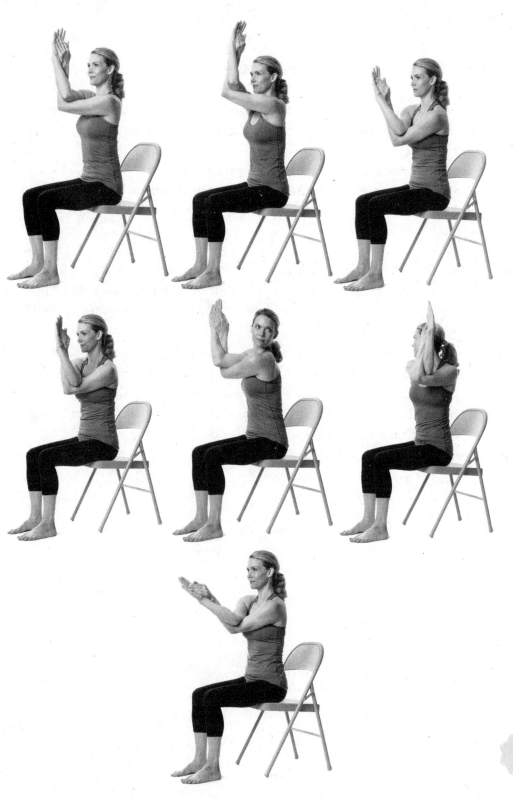

Cow Face Arms

Cow face arms is wonderful for balancing out our right and left sides; stretching the arms, shoulders, and wrists; and relieving tension and tightness in the triceps.

Works Your: Arms (especially the triceps), hands, and wrists

Try This: When you notice you're overusing your dominant hand; feel tension in the arms, shoulders, and wrists; or need to open up the chest and fronts of the shoulders

1. Sit tall with your feet hip-width apart and firmly on the floor, and with your hips toward the edge of the chair and your back straight. Take your right arm up overhead and bend the elbow so the palm rests between the shoulder blades.

2. Internally rotate the left arm and take it behind your back and slide the hand up toward the right hand. See if you can clasp the hands (you can also use a belt, tie, towel, or strap to help reach), or just keep the hands where they land and hold and breathe for 5 to 8 breaths. Make sure to bring your head back in line with your spine and continue sitting up straight.

3. Repeat on the opposite side.

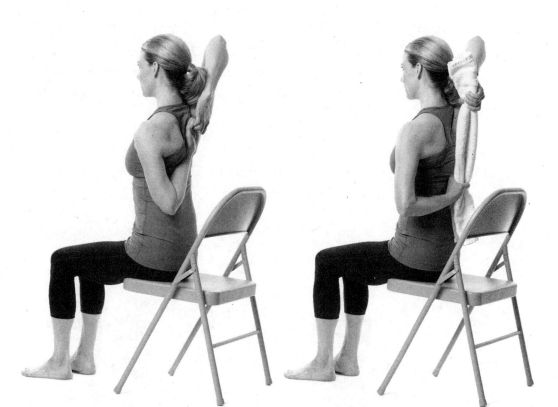

Have you ever noticed how different each side of your body is? This is especially true when it comes to our arms. I often find my right arm is much tighter in the front of the rotator cuff and I have more difficultly stretching it in certain poses.

Take cow face arms, for instance, which requires major rotation and flexibility in the rotator cuff. When I try to wrap my arm up behind my back, it is so much tighter on my right side than my left.

You may be right- or left-hand dominant and that side is definitely going to be tighter. Exercises like this one will start to bring the right and left sides into better balance.

High Altar Arms

This exercise involves a bit of imagination. It helps us reach up and allows ourselves to imagine something we truly want to bring into our lives. High altar arms also provides an amazing release in the wrists all the way down through the arms. By lifting your arms, you also raise the ribs and create space in the entire body.

Works Your: Arms, wrists, shoulders, and sides
Try This: When you want some relief in the arms, shoulders, and wrists, or need a little pick-me-up and positive energy in your life

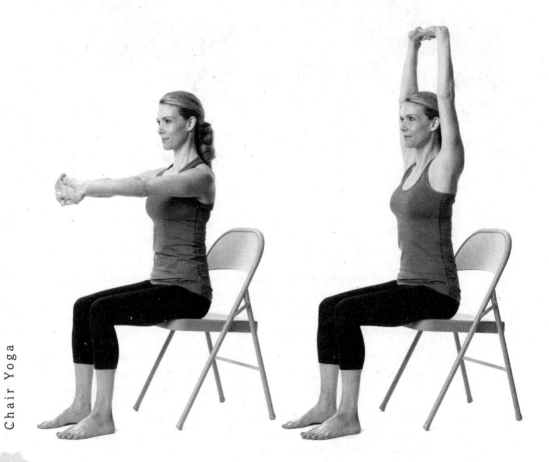

1. Sit tall with your feet hip-width apart and firmly on the floor, and with your hips toward the edge of the chair and your back straight.

2. Stretch your arms out in front of you, interlace the fingers and invert the palms so they face away from the torso. Take a few breaths here and feel how great this stretch is in and of itself.

3. Keep the ribs soft as you lift your arms up above your head, creating an altar above you. Make sure the tops of your shoulders remain down and stretch from elbow to wrist. Bring the elbows back in line with the ears as much as possible.

4. Envision something on top of the altar above you that you want to bring into your life. Hold for at least 5 to 8 breaths.

5. Release the arms and then repeat the posture, but try it with the opposite thumb in front by switching the way you clasp your hands. We often get stuck in habit and always hold our hands together the same way. By switching it up, it keeps our body and brain in the moment.

High Altar Triceps Presses

These triceps presses are an easy way to tone the arms while giving you an even deeper stretch.

Works Your: Arms, wrists, and shoulders
Try This: To tone the triceps region or for a good wrist and forearm stretch

1. Starting in high altar arms pose (see page 76), bend the elbows to the sides and then straighten the arms back up to the ceiling. Every time you bring the arms down, bow your head forward slightly and imagine bringing that gift in to yourself, then offering it back up.

2. Repeat 5 to 8 times. Make sure to really keep the tops of the shoulders released down away from the ears as you press the elbows straight up again.

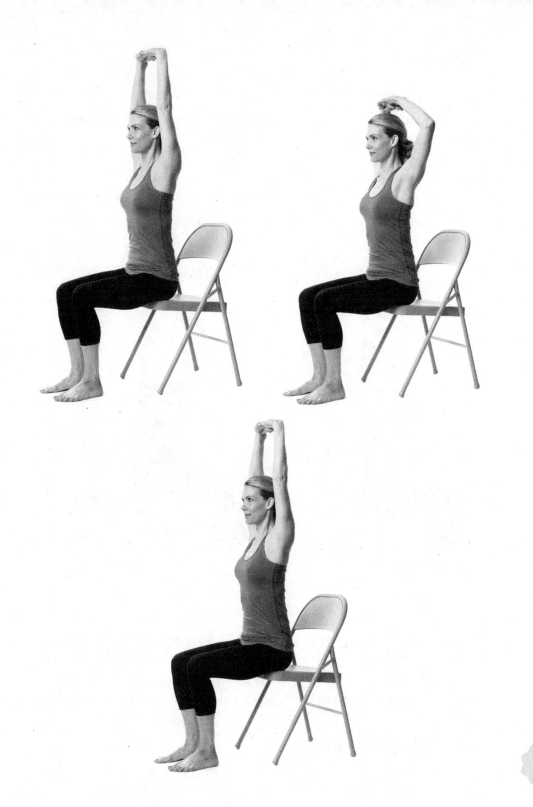

High Altar Leans

This exercise gives you an even deeper stretch through the entire arm and waist region and opens up the tops of the shoulders a little bit more.

Works Your: Arms and waist

Try This: To open up the lungs and feel the connection between the arms and the side body, or release tension in your shoulders and wrists

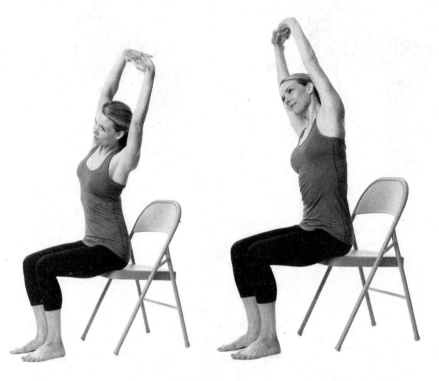

1. Starting in high altar arms pose (page 76), lean to your left as far as you can while still anchoring the right hip to the chair. Hold for five breaths, come up through the center, and then lean over to the right for five breaths. Think of moving up and over so you still keep length in the sides of the waist.

2. Repeat 2 to 3 more times on each side.

Side Leans with Wrist Pull

Side leans while pulling on the wrist to assist allow you to manually stretch your entire arm. It's like putting yourself on your own personal rack and really lengthening the muscles out to relieve the joints.

It can be a natural transition to add the wrist pull after you've done high altar leans or you may just want to do these any time you want to wake up your upper body.

Works Your: Arms, shoulders, and waist

Try This: First thing in the morning or whenever you need an energy boost

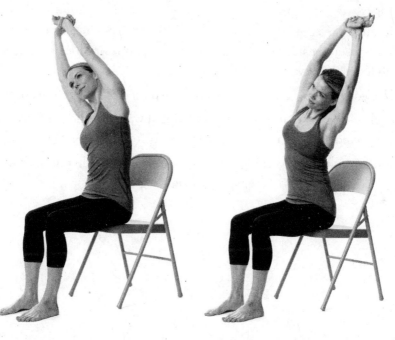

1. Sit tall with your feet hip-width apart and firmly on the floor, and with your hips toward the edge of the chair and your back straight. Lift your arms overhead and take hold of your left wrist with your right hand.

2. On an exhalation, pull yourself over to the right and concentrate on stretching the left arm out all the way down through the waist. Hold for 5 to 8 breaths.

3. Inhale back up to sit and repeat on the other side, holding your right wrist with your left hand.

Triceps Dips Using Seat of Chair

Who doesn't want toned arms? The back region of the arms starts to get loose and flabby when we don't exercise or tone it properly. Triceps dips are such an easy exercise to complete with a chair and the perfect thing to do on a daily basis to firm up the backside of the arms.

Works Your: Triceps, chest, shoulders, back, and abs
Try This: When you want to show off at work (just kidding!), need some toning (with a bonus ab workout), or need a metabolism boost

1. Sit tall at the edge of your seat with your feet hip-width apart. Place your hands on either side of your hips, with your palms wrapped around the seat and facing backward.

2. Slide your hips off the chair but keep the back close to the edge of the seat.

3. Bend your elbows and lower your hips toward the floor as you inhale. Exhale and lift back up to your starting position. Try for 15 to 20 dips.

4. For more advanced variations, extend both legs straight out in front of you or lift one leg up for ten reps, then switch legs.

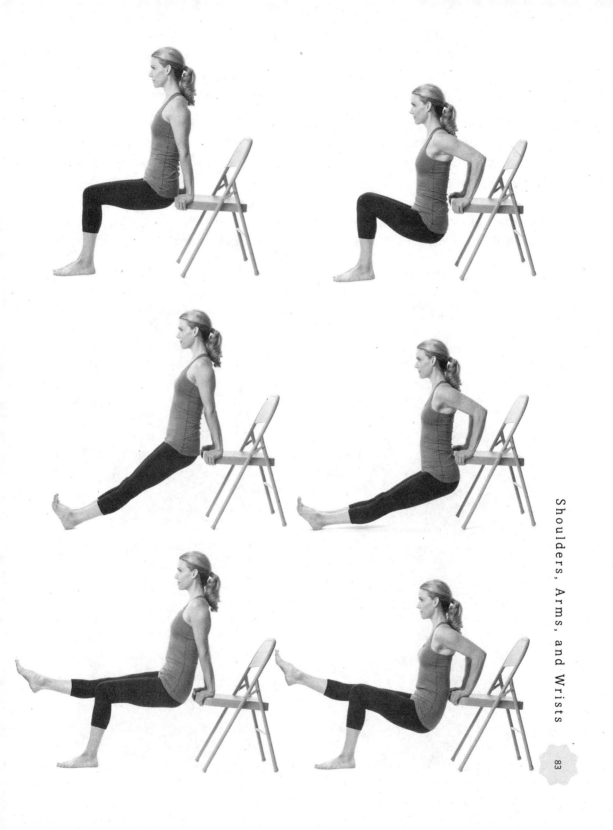

1-2-3-4 Wrist Workout

This exercise was first shown to me by a friend who was suffering from carpal tunnel; she said it worked wonders for her. Many of us suffer from wrist or hand issues or just want to prevent the onset of overuse injuries. I love how easy this exercise is and how much it forces our brain to focus.

Works Your: Wrists, hands, fingers, and brain
Try This: If you want to prevent or treat carpal tunnel syndrome, need some wrist and hand relief, or want to focus the mind

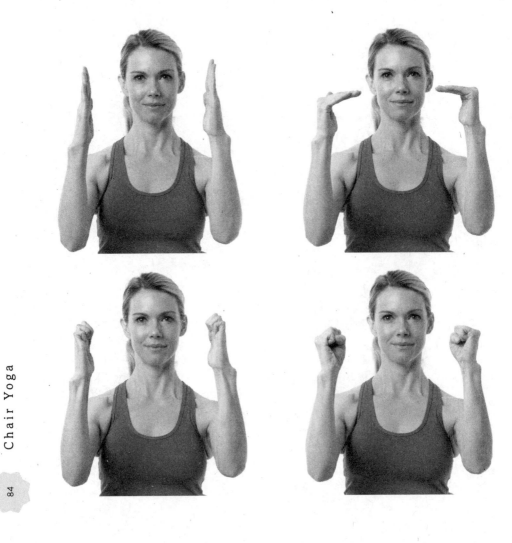

1. Start seated upright. Lift your arms out in front of you with your elbows bent and your palms facing each other.

2. Keep your hands straight and palms flat, then bend at the fingers so they are parallel to the floor, making a tent. Next pull the upper part of the fingers into the lower part of the fingers like claws, and finally shape and squeeze both hands into fists.

3. Repeat these four motions (straight, tent, claw, fist) twenty times.

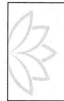

The next time you have the urge to check social media or wander off from your task at hand, try this exercise. It takes only five minutes and will refocus you, readying you to get back to work with a cleared mind and fresh hands.

Triceps Stretch

We don't realize how tight a muscle can be sometimes until we give it a good stretch. This is particularly true when it comes to our triceps. Since they are on the backs of the arms, we aren't as aware of these muscles. Tight triceps can lead to all sorts of issues from the elbows down into the hands. It's important to lengthen and release them when we can.

Works Your: Triceps, shoulders, and upper back

Try This: When you start to feel tightness in the elbow joint and back of the arm, feel like you could use a good front body opener, after your triceps dips (page 82), or as a prelude to a deeper stretch such as cow face arms

1. Start seated at the edge of your chair.
2. Lift your left arm up above you and bend the elbow overhead so the hand drops behind the head toward the left shoulder blade.
3. Take your right hand to the elbow and help pull the arm back farther into the stretch.
4. Hold for 5 to 8 breaths before switching sides.

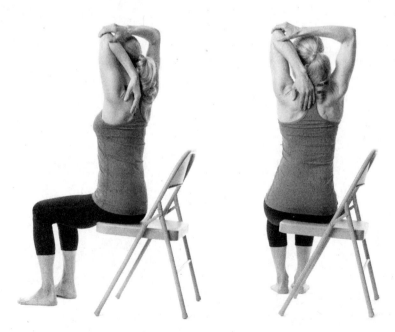

Behind-the-Back Opposite Elbow Hold

This simple pose is an instant posture improver! Forward head syndrome and poor posture are more prevalent than ever considering that many of us spend the majority of the day staring at a computer screen or down at our phones. Try this out and you'll feel the stretch across the front of your body and the opening of your rounded forward shoulders. You'll also feel more confident!

Works Your: Chest and spine

Try This: Whenever you find yourself slouching or rounding forward, have restricted breath, or have tension or tightness across the front of the body

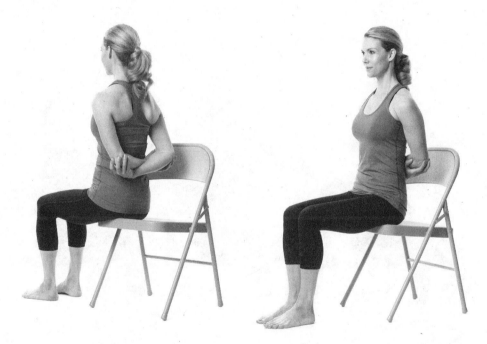

1. Start seated upright at the edge of your chair and take your arms around behind you. Try to hold on to opposite elbows.

2. Hold this position for 5 to 8 breaths. Try to do it again, but this time take the opposite arm on top.

Flipped Clasped Hands

This little clasped-hands flip of the wrists is another exercise/brain teaser. The movement of holding our hands with the wrists crossed and then flipping them through keeps our mind actively engaged in the movement. I find students especially get confused when they come back and work on switching to the opposite hand on top. This exercise really shows us just how tight we are in our forearms and wrists as well.

Works Your: Hands, forearms, and wrists
Try This: When you need some wrist relief, want to mix things up, feel stuck in the mind, or want a simple stretch but don't have much space

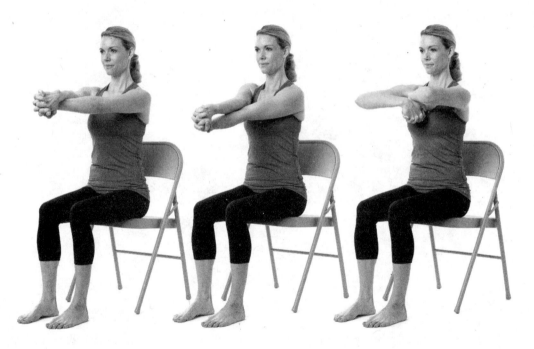

1. Start seated upright and stretch your arms straight out in front of you. Cross your arms at the wrists so the right hand is above the left hand, flip the palms to face each other, and clasp the hands.

2. Turn the clasped hands under toward the torso, then try to extend them once again forward so the wrists have rotated around and you feel a major stretch in the forearms and right wrist especially.

3. Unwind by coming back toward your torso and out in front again. Switch the hands so the left hand is now on top and do the same twist under and stretch forward action.

4. Try each side once again and see if there's any more give in either wrist. Hold the stretch for at least thirty seconds on each side.

Hand Pulls

Sometimes the simplest stretches feel the best, while also showing us just how tight our forearms, hands, and wrists are. Just like the flipped clasped hands exercise, this one keeps our mind focused and balances out our right and left hands. It's really nice to use our other hand to assist and feel how much pressure we can apply, but just enough to get a deep stretch without overdoing it to the point of tensing other places or holding our breath.

Works Your: Wrists, forearms, and hands

Try This: When you are anxious and waiting somewhere, need a little break from the computer or portable device you use, or feel achiness or cramping in the hands, forearms, or fingers

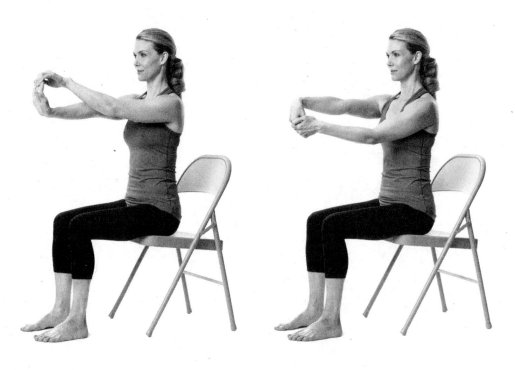

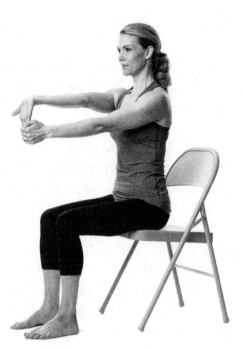

1. Sit up tall and stretch your right arm straight out in front of you with the palm facing out, so the hand looks like a "stop" gesture.

2. Take your left hand and pull the fingers of the right hand back toward the torso, holding for 30 to 60 seconds.

3. Now turn your right hand facing down and take the left hand over the top of the right hand. Press the back of the hand down, holding for 30 to 60 seconds.

4. Finally turn the right palm up to face the ceiling and use the left hand to pull the fingers down one last time for 30 to 60 seconds. Repeat everything on the left hand.

Behind-the-Back Prayer Hands

When you make prayer hands, either up or down your back (an easier modification), you're mentally telling yourself you've got your own back and you can handle anything coming your way. Cut yourself some slack and go slowly if it feels really intense.

Works Your: Pectoral muscles, shoulders, wrists, and forearms
Try This: When you need a boost of confidence, feel worried, or want some reassurance; need to open up your chest; want to stretch your arms, wrists, and hands; or could use an intense release

1. Sit tall with your feet hip-width apart and firmly on the floor, and with your hips toward the edge of the chair and your back straight.

2. Hold opposite elbows behind your back and then gradually work on pressing the palms together up between the shoulder blades. You can also do a prayer facing down the back to make it a little easier.

3. Really press the palms fully together and try to hold for 30 to 60 seconds if you can handle it. You can eventually work up to a few minutes and close your eyes as a little meditation.

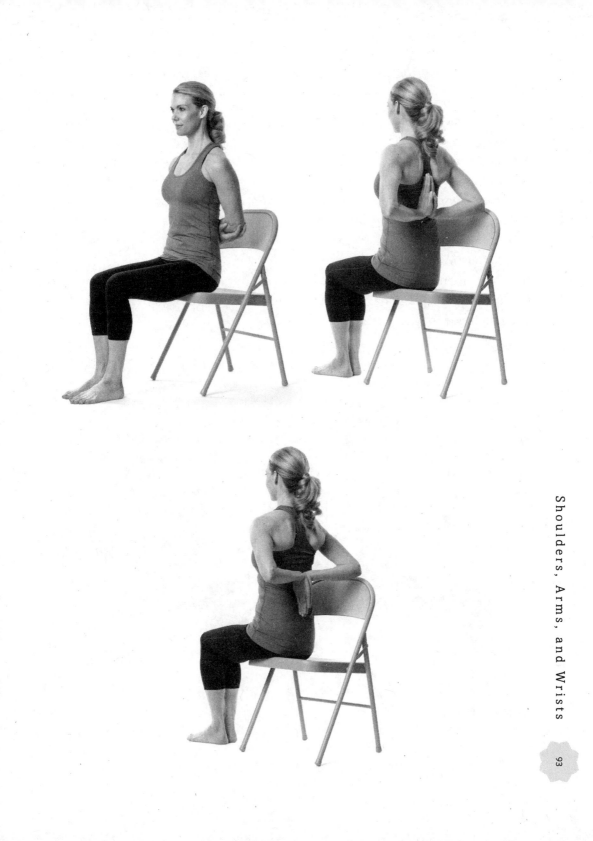

Behind-the-Back Clasped Hands

This is such a nice stretch to do any time of the day. I love to do it when I first wake up as I'm reading my e-mails and having my coffee, in the middle of the day when I need a refresh, or at the end of the day to just let it all go. When we clasp our hands behind our back we immediately lift open our chest and allow more oxygen in our lungs. I think of this exercise as automatic suspenders raising our chest up and dropping our shoulders down and back. It also provides great relief through the arms and shoulders.

Works Your: Wrists, arms, and shoulders

Try This: When you first wake up or arrive at your desk at work, need a midday break, find your energy flagging, need a reminder to breathe, or want to practice using both sides of yourself more evenly

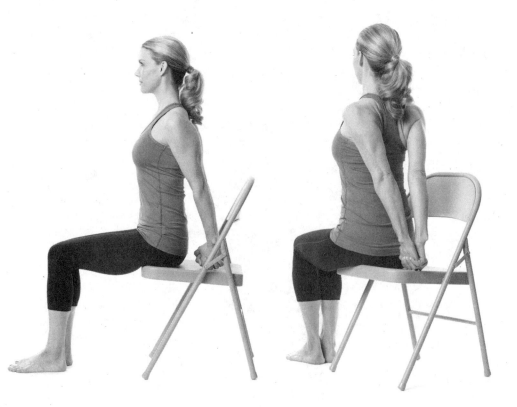

1. Sit tall with your feet hip-width apart and firmly on the floor, and with your hips toward the edge of the chair and your back straight.

2. Take the arms behind you and interlace the fingers. Keep the arms long and elbows extended as you squeeze the entire part of each palm together.

3. Lift your chest and open your heart as you breathe here for 5 to 8 deep, full breaths.

4. Release, relax for a second, and do it one more time with the opposite thumb on top.

It is so easy to fall into habit and lead with our one dominant side. When you start to make subtle changes like using the opposite thumb on top when you clasp the hands, you'll find you're more aware and awake in every moment of life.

Try using your nondominant hand to brush your teeth at night, unlock your door, or even eat your meal.

Downward Dog Arms

A downward dog a day keeps the doctor away! Many of us barely have time to eat break-fast each morning, but the next time you sit down somewhere, just think: you might as well perform your downward dog right there.

Works Your: Upper body and shoulders

Try This: When you need a breather, feel a little stressed, want a big shoulder opener, want a little blood flow to the brain, or need a moment to yourself

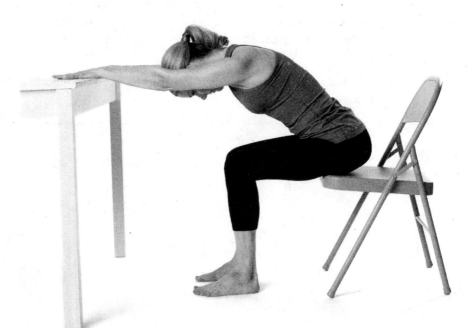

1. While seated at a desk or table, move the chair back far enough so you can lengthen your arms to the desk or table with only your palms flat on the surface. Make sure your arms are shoulder-width apart.

2. Press firmly into your palms as you let the upper body sway toward the floor. Keep the ribs drawn toward one another and the abdominals engaged.

3. Hold this downward dog desk variation for ten breaths.

6

Torso

The torso is our powerhouse! After years of practicing and teaching Pilates and yoga, I know how important this region of our body is. Here are some moves you can do to tone your abdominals, lengthen your spine, and strengthen your entire torso region.

Without a firm core, our spine is weak and our abs are weak and flabby, making us prone to back pain. Excessive sitting has been linked to excess body fat in the torso. Weight gain in the midsection puts us at risk of all sorts of issues, from herniated discs to type 2 diabetes, and has been linked with higher cortisol levels, elevated cholesterol levels, and a greater risk for heart attacks.

Our torso can also hold a lot of pent-up energy. Breathing deeply into the sides, lower back, front body, and waist can really make a difference in our mood and stamina. Some of my all-time favorite stretches involve the spine and torso region. Joseph Pilates's famous quote, "You're only as young as your spine is flexible," really holds true. The more we can tap into the energy in our core and use it to support our spine and torso, the younger we feel and the more energy we have.

So many postures require initiating the move or holding the move from the abdominals. Imagine you have a cylinder or straw rising up inside of you from the very base of your spine. Draw the energy up the center of the straw, starting at the pelvic floor and moving up through the transversus abdominis, stabilizing the entire body.

Your core muscles are the central link in a chain connecting your upper and lower body. Weak or inflexible core muscles can impair how well your arms and legs function. Whether you're hitting a tennis ball or sweeping the floor, the necessary movements originate or flow through your core.

So many activities depend on a strong core, from the simple act of bending to put on shoes, to most athletic endeavors, to housework, gardening, and even sex. Once you learn to engage your abdominals the right way, you'll find a natural lift and length without having to force anything. These exercises will help you gain strength in the core and freedom in the spine and torso so you can sit with ease and poise.

Your core muscles stabilize your body. Core exercises can improve balance and lessen your risk of falling. Weak core muscles also contribute to slouching and poor posture. Good posture trims your silhouette and projects confidence. More important, it lessens strain on the back and allows you to breathe deeply. A strong midsection and torso help us stay focused, lean, and healthy.

Engage Your Core

Keep your core engaged when performing all of these exercise and all yoga exercise for that matter. Our abdominals are endurance muscles and can be worked all the time. Here are some moves you can do to tone your abdominals, lengthen your spine, and strengthen your entire torso region. Make sure to use your ujjayi breath (page 8) and initiate each movement from your core.

Chair Twist

Twists are very beneficial for our spine and entire torso, and they really help us get a 360-degree view. I find twists are most helpful when I feel my energy flagging and need a refresh, or I have a sluggish digestive system and need some help getting things moving again. Twists lubricate the spine and open up our back, shoulders, and hips. They help us gain a new perspective and increase range of motion in the intervertebral discs.

Works Your: Spine, core, and oblique muscles
Try This: Whenever you want to gain some perspective around yourself, need a refresh, feel a little backed up, or want to whittle your waist

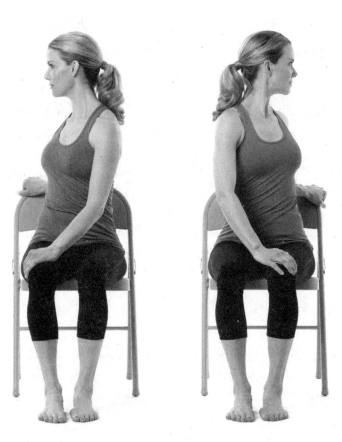

Chair Yoga

1. Sit tall with your feet hip-width apart and firmly on the floor, and with your hips toward the edge of the chair and your back straight. Take your right hand behind you to the top of the chair and your left hand to your right knee.

2. On an inhalation extend up through the spine, then on the exhalation twist deeper to your right. Continue to lift and twist for 5 to 8 breaths.

3. Come back to center and repeat on the other side.

4. Repeat 2 to 3 more times or throughout the day whenever you need a refresh.

Side-to-Sides

Moving laterally is something we aren't as accustomed to as moving forward and back. When our body is asked to move in new or different ways, it builds new neural connections in the brain and keeps us young. You may feel silly or uncoordinated doing this move at first, but keep practicing until you get the hang of it. To take it to the next level, try Side-to Sides with Waist (page 118).

Works Your: Obliques, core, waist, and lower back
Try This: Whenever you want to get some creative juices flowing, feel stiff or tight in your lower back region, need to focus, or want to tone your midsection

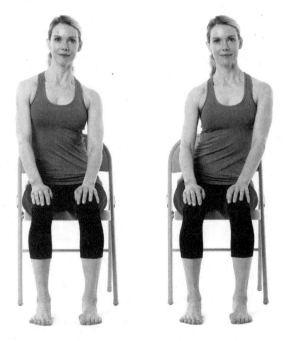

1. Sit tall with your feet hip-width apart and firmly on the floor, and with your hips toward the edge of the chair and your back straight.

2. Keeping your lower body and legs still, slide your rib cage to the right as you inhale.

3. On your exhalation move to the left side in the same way.

4. Try moving from side to side 15 to 20 times as fast or as slow as you would like to go.

Side Bends

The spaces between our hips and ribs can easily get compressed, especially after sitting for too long or slouching when we stand. Alongside our lower back on either side of the spine rest our kidneys. Our kidneys are like little battery packs that keep us energized. When we squash down on them all day long, we feel lethargic and spent. Opening up the sides with twists and side bends helps keep our kidneys juiced up and our body and mind charging all day long.

Works Your: Waist (including the love handles) and abs
Try This: For a longer, deeper stretch in the sides of the waist

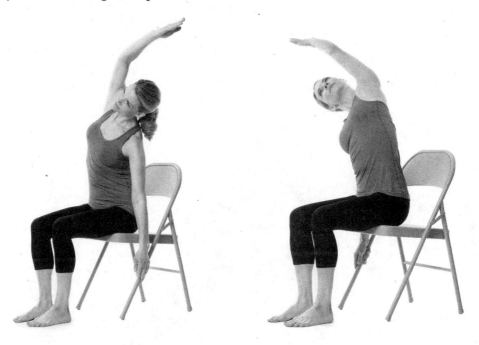

1. Sit tall with your feet hip-width apart and firmly on the floor, and with your hips toward the edge of the chair and your back straight. Inhale and lift your right arm up alongside your ear with the palm facing inward.

2. On your exhalation, start to slowly lean to the left. You can prop your left hand on the seat or let it hang by the outer left thigh.

3. Hold here for 5 to 8 breaths, going deeper into the side bend with each exhalation. Inhale to rise back up to sit and repeat on the opposite side.

Extended Side Angle

Extended side angle is a wonderful stretch that requires more space around you since you need to extend your legs open into a warrior II–type stance. Make sure you have the room, and work on really spinning the waist around toward the ceiling in this stretch.

Works Your: Hips, legs, and lower back

Try This: When you want to fully oxygenate the lungs, need to release the back, or want to feel more energized and strong

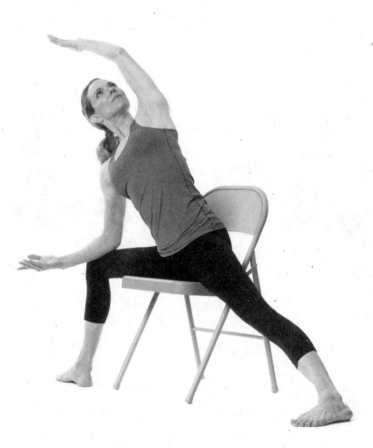

1. Sit at the edge of your chair and open your right knee to the side with the right foot turned out 90 degrees. Extend your left leg straight and angle your left foot in about 75 degrees. You're coming into a seated warrior II position.

2. From here, lay your right forearm on your right knee with the palm facing upward. Use the back of the arm to slide the knee more to the right. Extend the left arm up and alongside the left ear, overhead in the direction of the right knee.

3. Feel the length and reach from the outer left foot all the way through the left fingers. Hold for 5 to 8 breaths on the right side, come up to sit, and repeat on the left side. Repeat each side two more times.

Seat Lifts

How cool is it to work your abs while you're seated? By learning how to lift our seat up off the chair, we gain deep access to our innermost abdominals. It's also a good swift kick in the butt when we find we are stuck in our seat for too long. This exercise may seem a little challenging at first, but you can work your way up to the full movement.

Works Your: Transverse abdominals, pelvic floor muscles, and core region
Try This: For a good ab workout, or if you notice you're slumping or letting your belly hang out

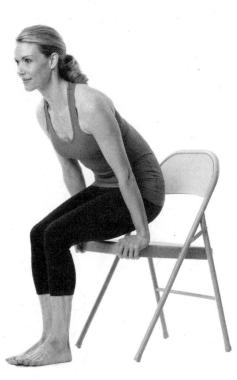

1. Sit tall with your feet hip-width apart. Place your hands on either side of your seat or toward the outer edges of your chair.

2. Relax for a second, then try lifting your butt up off the chair without using your legs as much as possible. Imagine your abdominals and arms lifting you up, and press your shoulders down away from your ears.

3. Hold for 1 to 2 seconds and lower down. Repeat up to ten times.

Seat lifts also tone your pelvic floor region and get your internal core all fired up. I love this exercise as a new mom and for postnatal women, but really everyone can benefit from it.

Scale Pose

Scale is a challenging pose that requires you to lift your entire seat and legs out of the chair. If it's too challenging at first, keep working the seat lifts (page 106) and the leg lifts (page 108) until eventually you can combine the two.

Works Your: Lower abdominals, pelvic floor muscles, entire core region, and arms
Try This: When you need a boost of energy, feel stuck in your seat for too long, or want to work the abs like nothing else

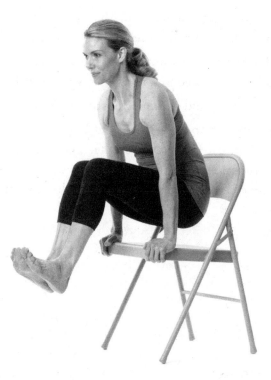

1. Sit at the edge of your seat and place your hands on either side of your hips with the fingers facing forward and wrapped around the seat of the chair.
2. Engage your core muscles, and on an inhalation press your hands down and lift your hips and legs up and try to hover for a second.
3. Lower down and repeat 2 to 3 more times.

Torso

Leg Lifts

Leg lifts are another great way to tone and strengthen the abdominals. These are a bit simpler than full-body lifts and can help with energy, restless leg syndrome, leg cramps, and even blood clotting when flying.

Works Your: Core, hip flexors, psoas, inner thighs, and pelvic floor muscles
Try This: When you are restless at work, on a plane, or in a waiting room; want to work your core; or need to focus

1. Sit at the edge of your seat and imagine a tight seat belt from hip rim to hip rim as you draw your lower abdominals in and upward.

2. From your abdominals, concentrate on lifting your right leg a few inches off the floor. Hold for two seconds and then lower the leg back down.

3. Repeat using the left leg, and alternate legs for 10 to 12 repetitions.

4. Next try lifting both legs up at the same time. You may need to lean slightly back in your chair or use your hands on the edge of the chair for support. Repeat 10 to 12 times. Try not to grip anywhere else in the body, but concentrate on using your core and torso to initiate the movement.

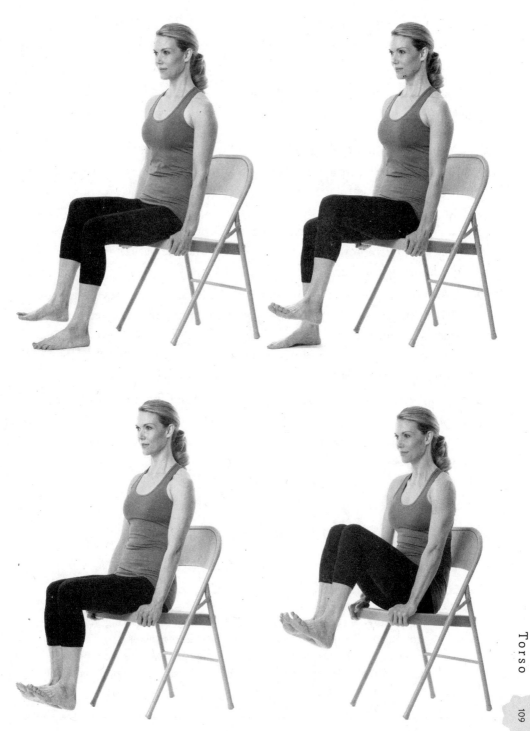

Leg Reaches and Leg Reaches with Twists

To amp up the abdominal work even more, you can incorporate leg reaches into your seated exercises. I personally use these with many of my clients and they feel their abs working right away.

Works Your: Abdominals, lower back, and legs
Try This: To work the entire abdominal region, when you want some cross-training, or when you find yourself slouching

1. Sit at the edge of your seat. Place both hands on either side of the chair with the fingers facing forward and wrapped around the base of the chair. Lift your knees up toward your chest.

2. Hinge the torso back enough to act as a cantilever and shoot your legs out straight, then draw them back in. Try going in and out for twenty repetitions. You'll need space in front of you, so make sure you have the room. You can modify it by lengthening the legs forward and slightly down, or just try to lengthen out a little bit before pulling the knees back in.

3. Next alternate shooting the legs out with pulling them toward the right shoulder in a twisting motion, then lengthen out and twist back in toward the left. Continue leaning from side to side in a twisting motion for twenty more repetitions.

Make sure to keep your core strong by imagining sucking your belly button to your spine so you don't feel this in the lower back. You may also get tight in the hip flexors when doing this exercise, so modify by keeping the knees slightly bent or focus on using the abdominals, not the legs, to initiate and control the movement.

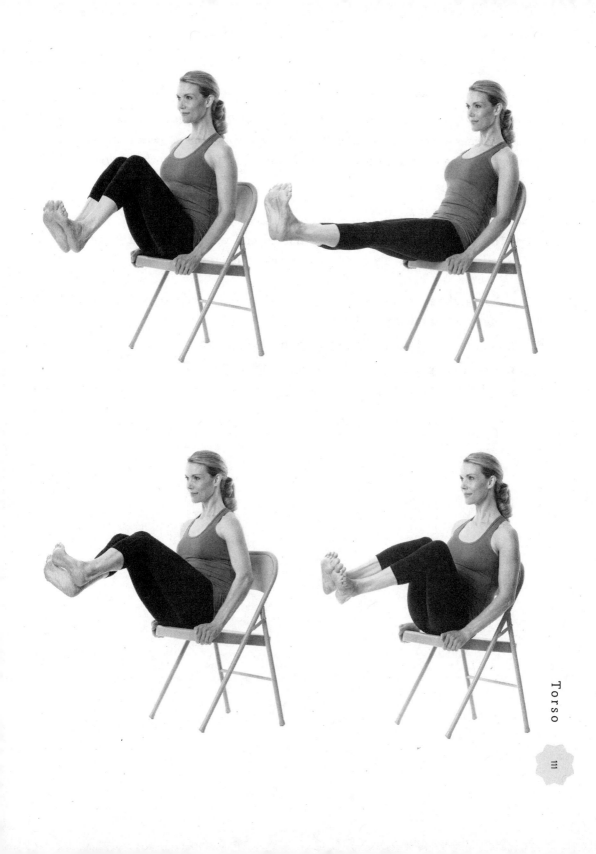

Bicycles

Bicycling the legs is always a great way to engage the abdominals and work the lower body. I also love this exercise for the brain. When we put our mind in our muscle, we get better results. Bicycling the legs requires coordination and focus (especially when we reverse the movement).

Works Your: Inner thighs, lower abs, obliques, core, and legs
Try This: When you feel yourself distracted and unfocused, want to tone and strengthen the abdominals, or have extra pent-up energy to release

1. Start at the edge of your chair with hands on either side of your hips, holding on to the outer part of the seat.
2. Engage your abdominals and lift your legs up in front of you.
3. Pedal the legs forward for twenty repetitions.
4. Pedal the legs backward for twenty repetitions.

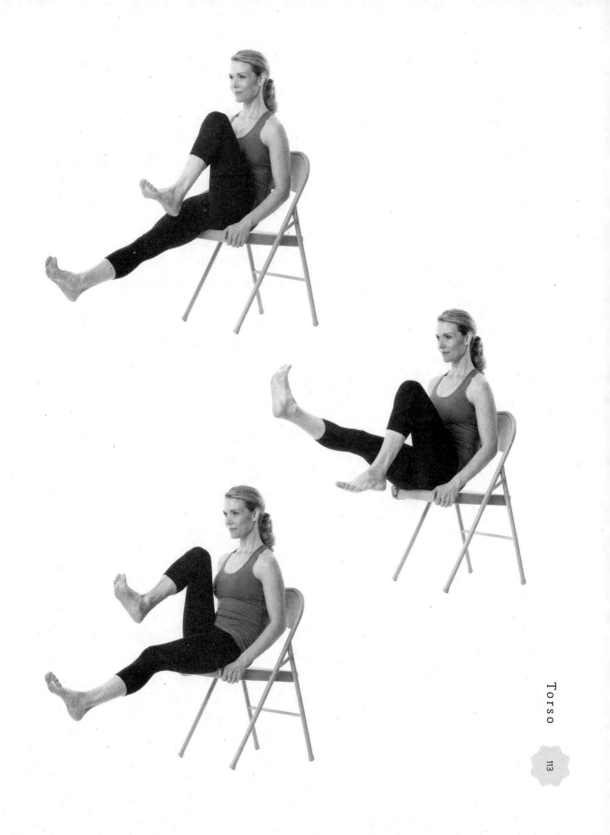

Single Leg Stretch

Now that you're really firing up your core and working your abs, you can experiment with different chair abdominal exercises. One of my favorite things to do when I'm at the airport is core work in the chairs. I can easily throw in some abdominal toning before boarding and it reminds me to stay lifted and keep my abs engaged when I'm flying. These moves can be done anywhere and at any time.

Works Your: Abs, legs, inner thighs, and pelvic floor muscles

Try This: When you want to strengthen and tone your abs, need some back support, want some extra energy, or have been sitting still for way too long (while watching TV, perhaps?)

1. Start seated toward the edge of your chair. Place the hands on the seat for support.

2. Lift your legs up in front of you with your knees bent and abdominals engaged.

3. Extend one leg straight out as you pull the opposite knee closer to your chest.

4. Repeat with the other leg.

5. Continue for twenty repetitions.

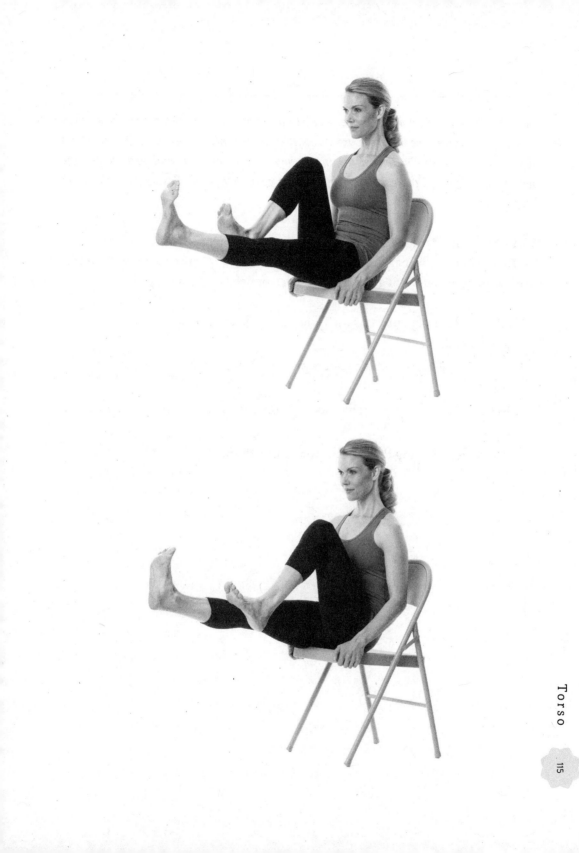

Scissors

For an advanced abdominal exercise, you can try scissors. Scissors is more intense than single leg stretch because both legs are straight the entire time, which makes the lever load greater. You have to really concentrate on drawing the abdominals in and up to support the lower back. If you find there's too much strain on your back or hip flexors, keep the knees slightly bent.

Works Your: Inner thighs, abs, lower back, and entire core

Try This: When you want a killer abdominal workout, have space to move your legs freely in front of you, want an extra challenge, or need some energy

1. Sit at the edge of your chair with your hands on either side of the hips, holding the seat.
2. Lean back slightly and lift your legs up in front of you with knees bent to begin.
3. Extend the legs out straight and work on scissoring one higher than the other.
4. Alternate switching the legs for twenty repetitions.

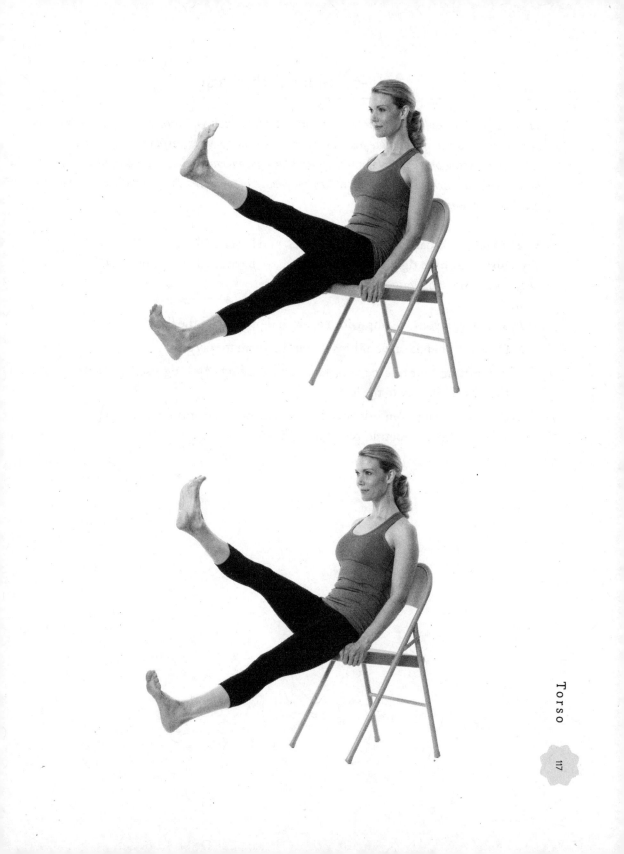

Side-to-Sides with Waist

This exercise is an isolation exercise and requires a lot of concentration and body awareness. When you can manipulate just one region of the body while keeping everything else still, you are truly practicing yoga. Every time we concentrate and connect our mind and breath with our movement, we find greater knowledge of ourselves and feel more confident in all areas of our life.

Works Your: Abs (particularly the obliques) and lower back
Try This: If you have tightness in the torso, have been stuck in one position for too long, like a good challenge, or need to concentrate

1. Sit tall with your feet hip-width apart and planted on the floor.
2. Place your hands on your hips to remind them to stay still.
3. Try shifting your ribs to the right without moving anything else. Then shift the ribs all the way to the left.
4. Continue going from side to side while keeping the entire body still for a series of twenty repetitions (ten to each side).

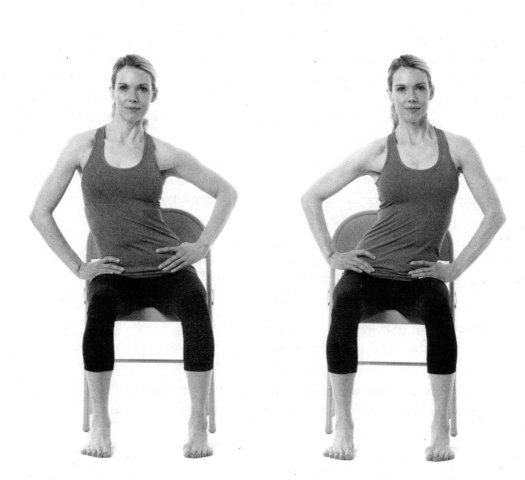

Try not to get discouraged if at first you can't do this or any exercise for that matter. Yoga is a lifelong process and it's easily accessible at any time, especially when done in a chair. Just know you have the tools to make your mind, body, and spirit feel better at any moment throughout your day.

Goddess Circles

In yoga class, we often come into a pose called the goddess squat. I love this position for bringing blood flow to the pelvis and firing up the inner thighs and lower abdominals. I have to admit, though, it's a pretty brutal pose to hold and quite taxing on the legs. What's so great about doing goddess squat in a chair is it takes the pressure off our legs and lets us focus on our core. If you're overworked at a desk all day long, these goddess circles are just what the doctor called for.

Works Your: Pelvic floor muscles, lower abs, and lower back

Try This: If you need some help toning the pelvic floor muscles, want to free up the torso, or want some extra toning in the sides, waist, and core region

1. Sit at the edge of your chair and widen your legs to either side of the seat with both feet turned slightly out.

2. Hold this position for 5 to 8 breaths.

3. Next place your hands on your knees and use your abdominals to start circling the torso around in a clockwise position. Make it really juicy and flowing to get the oblique muscles and core involved in the movement.

4. After about 15 to 20 circles in this direction, stop and go the other way. You can continue alternating each direction for as long as feels good.

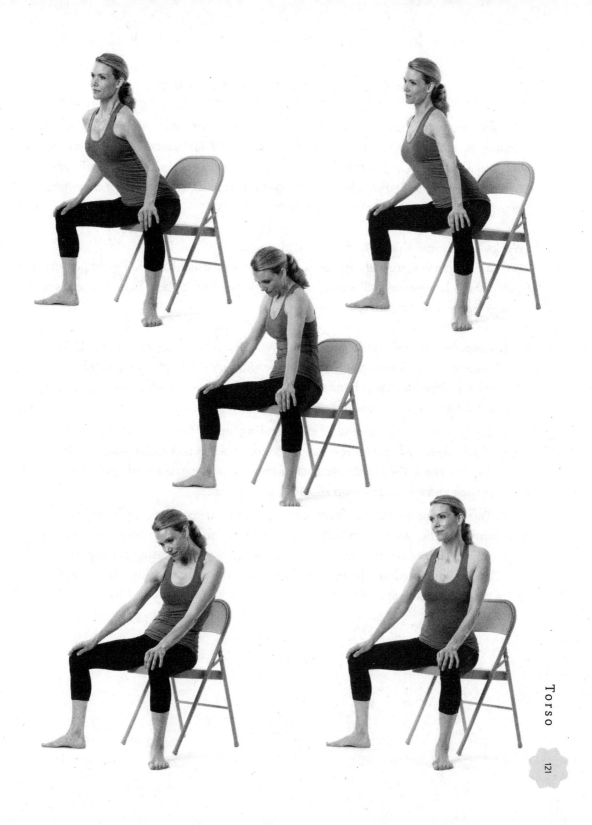

Goddess Side Stretch and Twist

Now that you've tapped into your inner goddess, try some of these variations in goddess position. So many of us suffer from tight inner thighs and hip flexors, which can keep us from using the core to its fullest power. Goddess supported in a chair automatically gives us a tactile aid to feel our pelvic floor muscles and open up our tight groins. We can engage our transverse abdominals so much easier in this position.

Works Your: Inner thighs, abdominals, and waist

Try This: When you are feeling creative, are pre- or postnatal (this is a great posture for moms-to-be and postdelivery once the doctor gives the green light to exercise), or need some soothing energy

1. Keep the same goddess leg position as you did in goddess circles (page 120). Place your left forearm on your left knee (or modify by placing your elbow on your knee) and side bend to the left. Hold for five breaths, come up, and repeat on the opposite side.

2. Try this again, but instead of side bending, open up the top arm to twist. If you're really flexible, you can place the other hand on the inside of the foot or even to the floor. Hold for five breaths or longer until you get a great stretch and feel you've worked the torso and waist.

3. This is one of my all-time favorite stretches, and if you are really bendy, you can take the top arm up and around behind your back to hold the upper-inner thigh of the bottom leg. Or play around with bending the top arm and placing the hand behind the head, then opening the elbow up toward the ceiling to deepen the stretch.

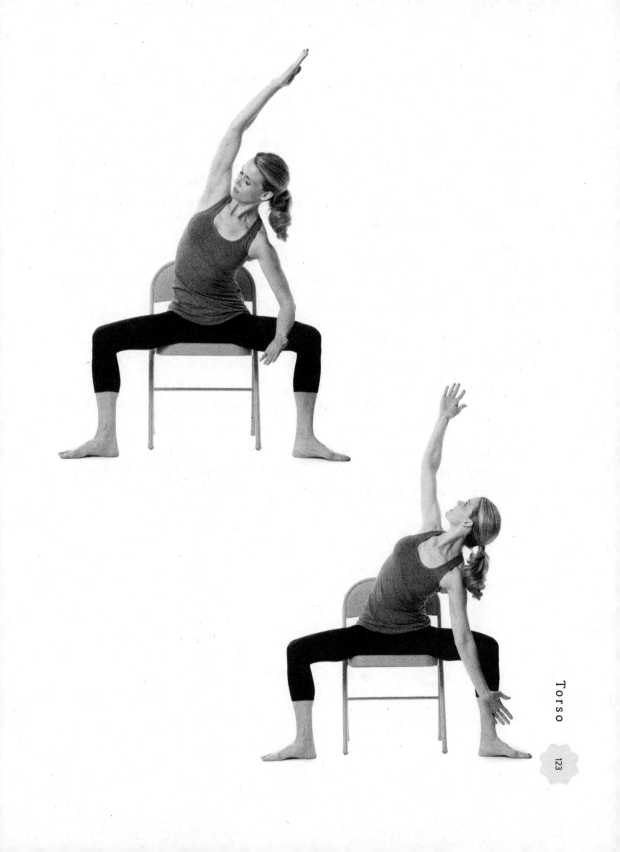

Side-to-Side Crunches with Hands Behind Head

When you really want some great waist whittling, try this awesome exercise. I often have my students do side-to-side crunches in straddle pose in class, and they inevitably have a hard time keeping their legs open and knees from falling inward. When you do this seated, you have the chair as a prop to help keep the knees and inner thighs open. You'll get your heart rate boosted and rev up your energy after this exercise. It's definitely one to help tone the love handles and trim the waist.

Works Your: Abs (particularly the obliques) and inner thighs
Try This: When you want to work your oblique and core muscles, have a hectic day, feel sluggish in the breath, or feel compressed in the waist

1. Start seated with your legs wide and feet slightly turned out. Place your hands behind your head with your elbows wide.

2. Inhale and lean toward your right leg, but keep your face forward (don't round in the upper back). As you exhale, bend all the way over to the left side.

3. Continue moving from side to side to work the abdominal muscles for twenty repetitions. You can go as fast or as slow as you want to go. Really concentrate on squeezing the waist as you lean from side to side.

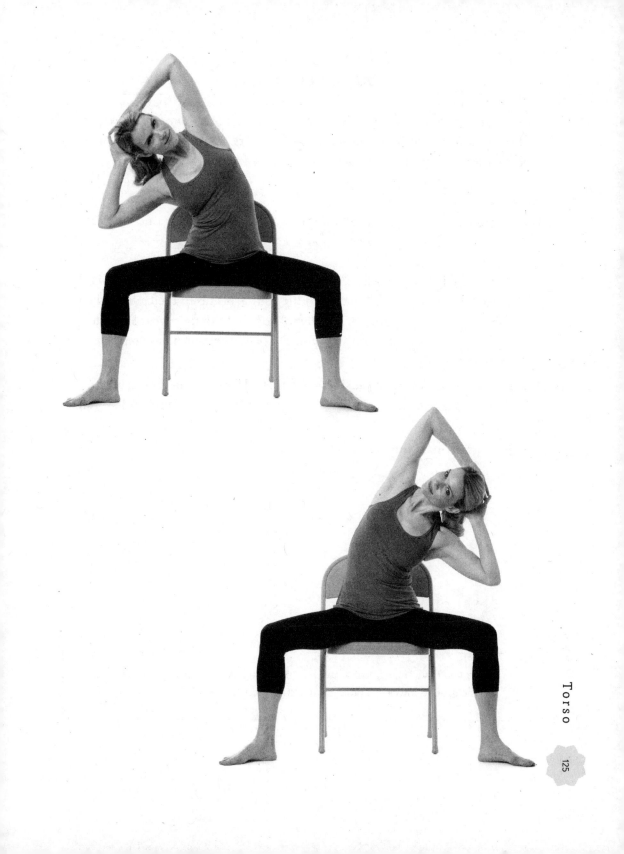

Straddle Forward Bend

After all the abdominal toning, it feels good to stretch it all out. Straddle forward bend lengthens the sides while still maintaining some core control. This pose is one of my favorites for feeling the weight of the world release from the entire body.

Works Your: Inner thighs and abdominals
Try This: After you've done your abdominal workout, if you feel drained or stressed, or if you have tension in the torso region

1. Sit at the edge of your chair with your legs wide. Turn your feet forward or slightly pigeon-toed. Inhale and lift your arms up to the ceiling, then exhale and fold forward, placing your hands on the outer edges of your feet or the floor, or, if you're too stiff, you can place them on a desk or table in front of you.

2. Let the torso release and the sides stretch. Hold for 8 to 10 deep, full breaths. Come back up to sit tall and feel the difference in your posture and overall well-being.

3. Repeat two more times.

Once you have this stretch down, try sitting up tall and lifting your legs up off the ground into a straddle for an extra torso challenge.

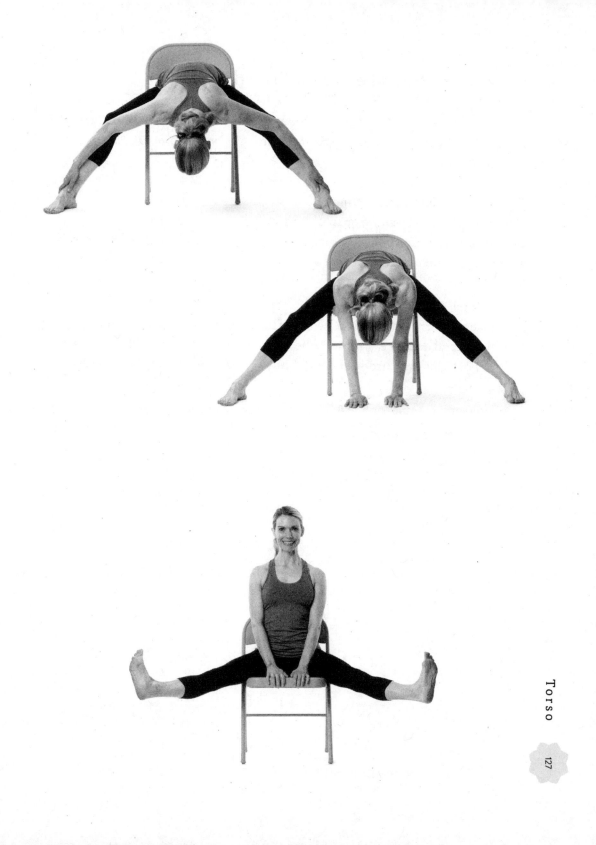

Straddle Forward Bend with Twist

To finish up the series, or to just add a bonus stretch, you can twist while you're in straddle forward bend. Now you're stretching the sides and waist long and working the core to initiate a great twist.

Works Your: Waist, core, and inner thighs

Try This: When you want to open up and stretch the entire torso, want to open up the lungs, feel stuck in your thinking or work, need some abdominal toning, or are a little backed up in your digestive system

1. Sit in straddle position and fold forward.
2. Place your right hand in the center of both legs directly under your head (if your hand doesn't easily touch the floor, you can place it on a block or stack of books, or even use your desk). Lift your left arm up to twist toward the ceiling.
3. Hold and breathe for 5 to 8 breaths, then switch arms.
4. Try each side one or two more times.

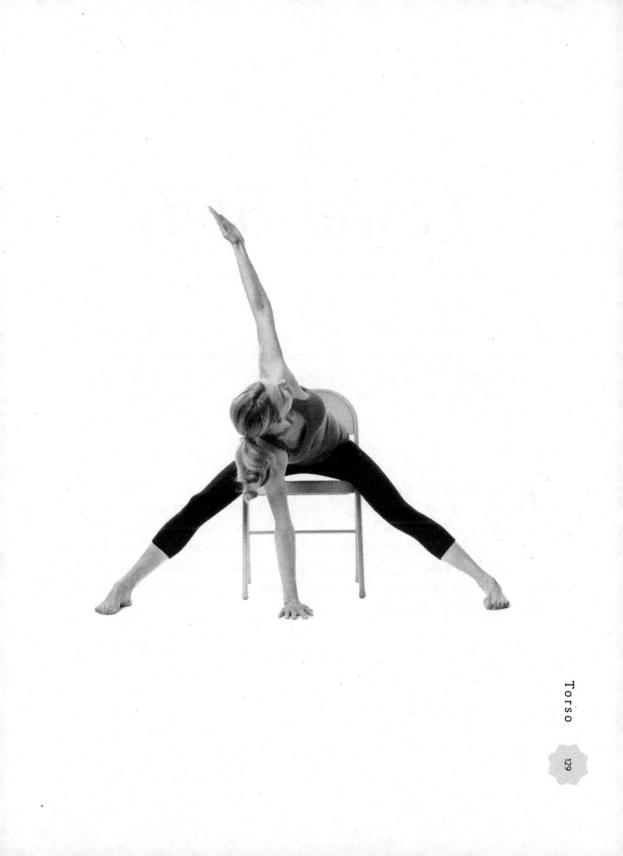

7

Lower Body

These are some of the most crucial chair exercises you can learn and incorporate into your daily practice. They will help keep your lower body strong and flexible and take the pressure off your lower back and vertebrae.

A lot of my students (especially women) ask me how to tone and tighten those trouble spots in the lower body region. Let's face it: sitting on our butt all day long gives us a flat ass! But you can do something about your rear by incorporating these awesome chair yoga poses and exercises. Doing simple stretches and strengthening moves will help you lengthen and lean out the hips, thighs, and love handle region. You'll also free yourself from lower back pain and feel so much better throughout your day.

There are many perks to doing yoga for the lower body. Our buttocks and thighs are our largest muscles and strengthening them gives our metabolism a nice boost. A majority of the people in Eastern cultures sit in a squat position, as opposed to in a chair, all day long. They rarely have hip and knee issues because those joints are forced through a full range of motion and the long leg muscles are constantly being stretched.

The people I meet who tell me, "I can't do yoga—my hamstrings are too tight," or "I can't touch my toes," are endless! I have so many students and beginners ask me how they can stretch the backs of their legs. First of all, we need to remind ourselves that yoga is a process, not a destination. On our road to more flexibility, it takes dedicated time, awareness, and breath to continue to open up. Also, we do many activities that create tightness and tension, so just like brushing our teeth, we need to repeat the practice over and over again to remove any buildup. And when we are consistent, we start to see amazing results and increased flexibility. We also learn to open up properly by engaging our abdominals and breathing deeply into each pose.

Our feet are rarely paid any attention, and giving them some TLC throughout the day makes a world of difference in our health and well-being. Our feet are our foundation, and learning how to use them properly, and stretch and strengthen them daily, can help correct postural imbalances, plantar fasciitis, cramping, and even bunions.

Get Ready for Lower Body Relief

Start with the feet and work your way up through the lower body. When you give your feet some attention, you also remind yourself to take a break, take a load off, and pamper yourself.

Feet

You can do all of these exercises in shoes, but they will be even more effective if you can do them in socks or, ideally, barefoot. You will want to be able to stretch your toes out completely. Most yogis practice barefoot so they can feel the movements from the ground up. Our feet help us with balance, stability, and mobility. Having agile, flexible feet and ankles can make a difference in all the movements we do. You can practice these foot exercises sitting at the edge of your seat or even in a more relaxed position, which makes them ideal for doing on the couch.

Foot Circles • Point/Flex

Toe Taps • Heel Raises

Squeeze/Spread • Alphabet

Foot Circles

Circling the feet and ankles helps with mobility in the ankle joints and relieves tension, as well as strengthens the tibialis muscles (front of shins).

Works Your: Ankles and lower leg
Try This: At the end of a long day when your feet need some relief

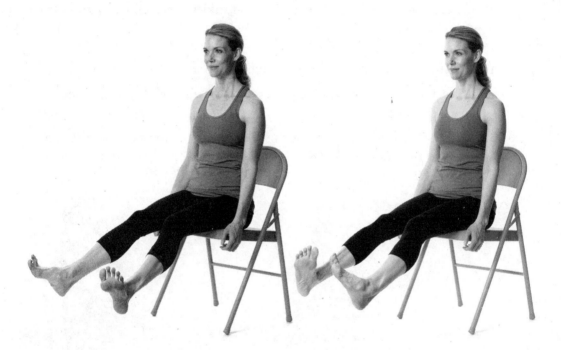

1. Sit at the edge of your seat or in a relaxed position.
2. Start with your right foot and circle the foot clockwise ten times, then circle the foot counterclockwise ten times. Make sure to keep the breath steady and even while doing the exercise.
3. Repeat with the left foot.
4. Try both feet at the same time if you want more of a challenge.

Point/Flex

It feels really good to articulate through the feet and ankles. We often wear unsupportive shoes and we really need to make sure our feet and ankles are strong and flexible. Pointing and flexing the feet is a good way to strengthen the feet and ankles and helps warm up the calves and shins.

Works Your: Ankles, calves, and shins
Try This: To stretch and strengthen the feet and ankles or work out any kinks from uncomfortable shoes

1. Sit at the edge of your seat or in a relaxed position.
2. Inhale and point your toes forward, then exhale and pull your toes back. Repeat ten times.
3. Repeat this series again, except this time inhale as you flex the feet and exhale as you point the feet.

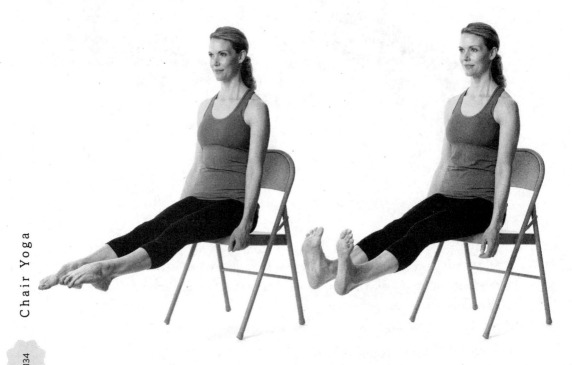

Toe Taps

Toe taps are great for those who have shin splints. I also often find myself tapping my toes when I need to release pent-up energy. Fidgeting throughout the day has been shown to increase metabolism and burn more calories.

Works Your: Ankles, shins, and feet
Try This: To relieve shin splints, increase your energy burn, or stimulate the brain

1. Sit at the edge of your seat or in a relaxed position.
2. Tap the toes up and down while keeping the heels on the floor. Always remain conscious of the breath and your posture while doing the taps.
3. Try tapping one foot at a time for ten reps, then the other, and then both. Or play around with tapping fast or tapping slow.

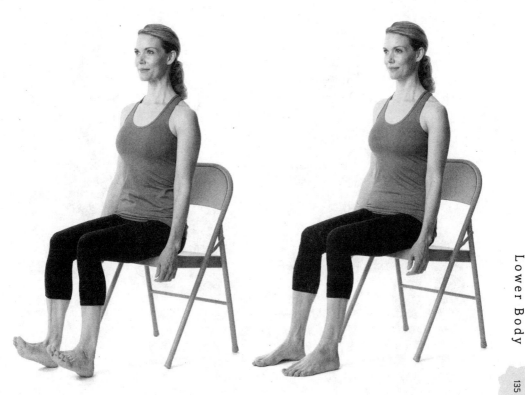

Heel Raises

To work the opposite side of the foot and the lower leg, you can try heel raises. Heel raises create range of motion in the ankle joint and lift our moods.

Works Your: Calf muscles and inner thighs
Try This: When you need a positive boost, want to strengthen your calves, or need to release nervous energy

1. Sit at the edge of your seat or in a relaxed position.
2. Lift and lower the right heel ten times, then lift and lower the left heel ten times. Lift and lower both heels ten times.
3. Repeat the entire sequence as many times as you would like. You can also alternate the heels and play around with the speed.

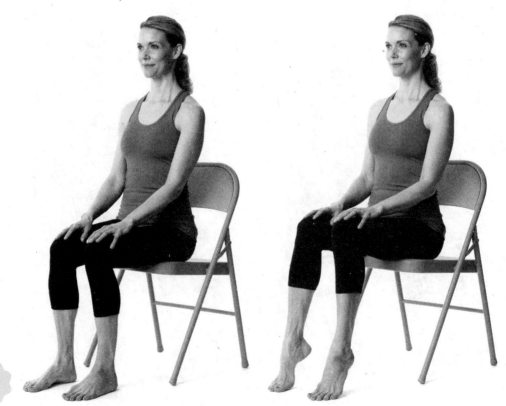

Squeeze/Spread

We often cram our feet into shoes that keep the toes all bunched together. This exercise of squeezing and spreading open the toes really helps you to work the little muscles between the toes and open them up. Notice where it's hard to open up and keep working on it.

Works Your: Toes, feet, and ankles

Try This: When you need some relief in the feet, have worn tight shoes or high heels, want to work on the range of motion in your toes, or need to prevent the onset of a bunion, corn, or other common toe issues

1. Sit at the edge of your seat or in a relaxed position.

2. Squeeze your toes as tightly as you can and hold for a second.

3. Spread the toes as wide as you can and hold for a second. Work on getting even your pinkie toe to separate from the fourth toe.

4. Repeat squeezing and spreading the toes at least ten times, eventually building up to twenty repetitions.

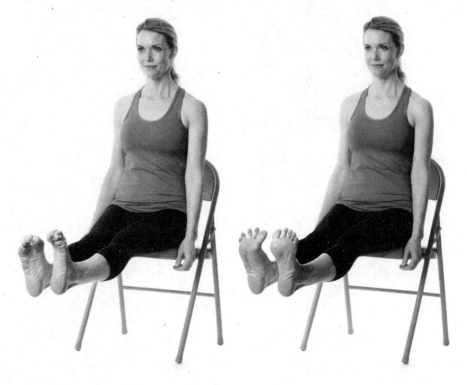

Alphabet

Tracing the alphabet with your foot (especially with your nondominant side) is wonderful for concentration as well as flexibility and mobility in the ankle joint and foot.

Works Your: Feet and ankles

Try This: When you have a tough problem to solve and need a break, are getting ready for your yoga practice and want to warm up your foundation, are watching television, or are prone to leg cramps at night

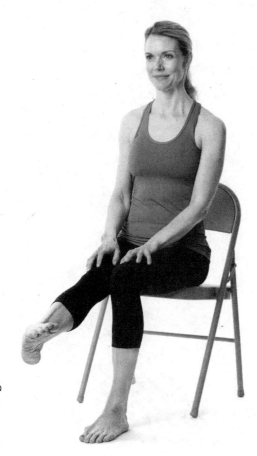

1. Sit at the edge of your seat or in a relaxed position.
2. With your right foot, trace the entire alphabet in the air.
3. Repeat with the left foot.
4. Keep your breath steady. Notice how energized your feet and mind feel.

Hips

Our hips are like the basement of our house: we often store a lot of energy and pent-up stress in them and continue to ignore the junk in the trunk until we are in pain or finally commit to some deep cleaning. Our hip joints are similar to our jaw joints and we can often clench them too tight. When you start to release the tension in your hips, you feel a world of difference in your back and posture. You will also strengthen weak hip muscles with some of these poses—tight muscles are often weak. Try practicing these lower body moves and stretches 3 to 4 times a week.

Ankle to Knee • Advance Ankle to Knee

Eagle Legs • Cow Legs • Butt Squeezes

Warrior I • Warrior II • Warrior III

Lunge • Goddess Squat

Ankle to Knee

This posture helps to ease tight outer hips and inner thighs. Ankle to knee is easy to do through-out the day and especially good for athletes who get super tight in their gluteal muscles.

Works Your: Outer hips, glutes, and inner thighs
Try This: To relieve tension in the hips and buttocks, if you're feeling lower back discomfort, or when you've been sitting in one position for too long

1. Sit tall at the edge of your seat.

2. Place your right ankle over your left knee with the right knee opening to the side.

3. Fold forward, placing your forearms across your calf until you feel a stretch in the outer right hip and thigh. Hold for 5 to 8 breaths. For a deeper stretch, let your arms fall at your side and round your torso forward completely.

4. Repeat on the opposite side.

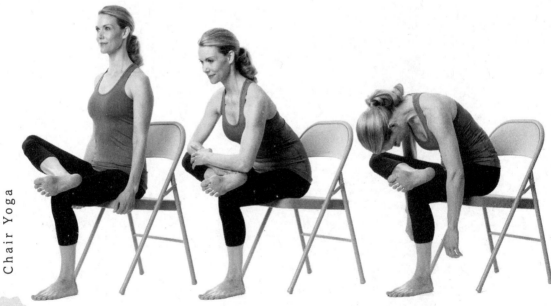

Advanced Ankle to Knee

If you've mastered ankle to knee pose, you can try elevating the legs to get a deeper stretch and work the core. Advanced ankle to knee is a great pose for the hips and deep external rotators. I like to perform this stretch when I'm on a long flight. For those of you with stiff or injured knees, be mindful of any pulling on the outer or inner knee as you do this stretch. If you feel too much strain, return to ankle to knee pose.

Works Your: Outer hips, buttocks, inner thighs, and abs

Try This: For a good deep stretch in the butt, for stiff legs, or to boost your energy

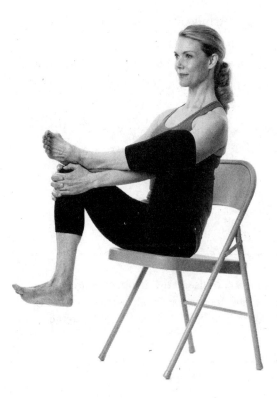

1. From ankle to knee pose on the left side, thread your left arm between your right leg and left leg and bring your right arm around on the outside. Use both hands to hold on to the right knee.

2. Lift both legs up off the floor and try drawing them up toward your chest without sinking in the lower back. Hold for 5 to 8 breaths.

3. Repeat on the opposite leg.

Eagle Legs

Eagle is said to be a pose that helps build focus. I also have a teacher who believes it helps prevent or diminish cellulite and varicose veins. I like to squeeze my legs tight and imagine crushing any self-doubt when I do this pose. Once I release from each side I have a new burst of stamina, enthusiasm, and focus.

Works Your: Legs, especially the inner thighs and calves

Try This: When you are losing focus (like in a long, tedious meeting), you want to tone and tighten the lower half, or you feel anxious

1. Sit tall with your feet hip-width apart and firmly on the floor, and with your hips toward the edge of the chair and your back straight.

2. Cross your right leg over your left and try to double cross the right foot behind the left ankle. If you can't reach, simply touch the right toes to the floor on the outside of the left foot.

3. Sit upright and draw your abdominals in and up. Keep your shoulders down and back, arms resting along your sides; or for an extra stretch add eagle arms.

4. Hold for 5 to 8 breaths and repeat on the opposite side.

Eagle legs is something you can also do discreetly, as people may just think you're crossing your legs! Bonus: Incorporate eagle arms (page 72) from chapter five ("Shoulders, Arms, and Wrists") if you want to do the entire pose.

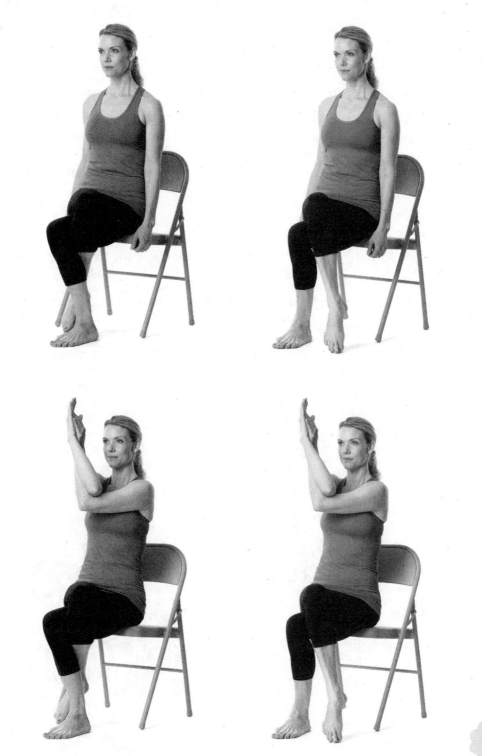

Cow Legs

Cow legs pose is another great hip opener and can be done in a chair as well as on the floor. I sometimes find I get an even deeper stretch when I do this in a chair.

Works Your: Inner and outer thighs
Try This: To bring some circulation to the legs, for a good butt stretch, or if your hips or lower back are bothering you

1. Cross your left leg over your right leg.
2. Lean back until you can lift your legs up and hold the front of the outer ankles.
3. Stay and breathe for 5 to 8 breaths, then switch sides.
4. Repeat 2 to 3 more times.
5. If leaning back is too complicated, you can modify by crossing your legs and leaning forward to feel the stretch in your outer hips.

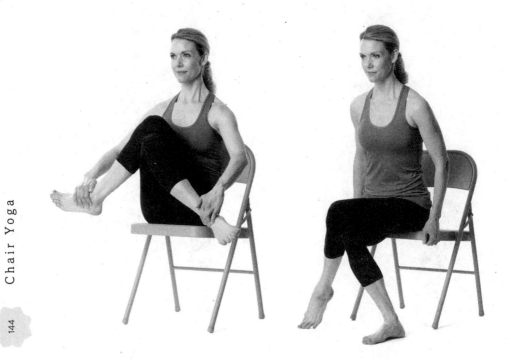

Butt Squeezes

This exercise is a good reminder that although we are seated, we can still give our butts a good lift. Our buttocks are actually part of our core as well, and the stronger they become, the more stable we are in our entire lower half. It's time to eliminate pancake rears once and for all and build up our backsides!

Works Your: Buttocks, pelvic floor muscles, and inner thighs
Try This: When you want to add a little lift to your rear end, need a boost in energy, or need to release pent-up tension in the hips

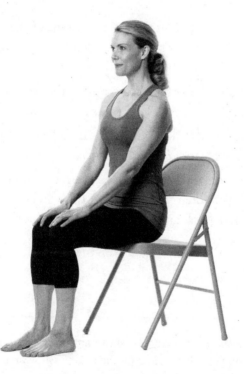

1. Sit tall with your feet hip-width apart and firmly on the floor, and with your hips toward the edge of the chair and your back straight.

2. Squeeze your buttocks together as if to lift up off the chair. Hold for two seconds and then release.

3. Repeat for twenty squeezes. Aim for three sets.

Warrior I

Warrior poses are some of the best lower body strengtheners and they build so much confidence. To perform the warrior poses with a chair, you need to really focus on contracting the muscles so you can benefit from each stance. Warrior poses stretch and strengthen the outer hips and buttocks, as well as the quadriceps, hamstrings, and inner thighs.

Works Your: Hips, buttocks, and thighs

Try This: Whenever you need some confidence, are feeling shaky or unsteady, or want to boost your lower half

1. Start seated with your butt at the left front edge of the chair, so you can sit on your right side and extend your left leg off the chair and back behind you.

2. Straighten through the left leg as you press the outer edge of the left foot into the floor. Make sure your left foot is angled forward 45 to 75 degrees.

3. Place your hands on your hips and try to direct them forward; you will feel a great stretch in the front of the left psoas, quadriceps, and hip flexor.

4. Keep your hands on your hips or place them on your desk if you have one in front of you. For added difficulty, lift the arms up and press the palms together overhead. Look up toward the hands.

5. Hold for 5 to 8 breaths. Repeat on the opposite leg. Try each side 2 to 3 more times.

Virabhadrasana is the Sanskrit name for the warrior poses we practice in yoga. It's named for the soldier who barreled up through the floor of the castle to save his princess from her father, the evil king, who had no interest in her marrying a foot soldier.

This is the first pose he performed, with his arms overhead pressing up toward the ceiling above him (the castle floor). We often have our own ceilings above us and battles to fight. Warrior I gives us the confidence and willpower to press through any obstacles.

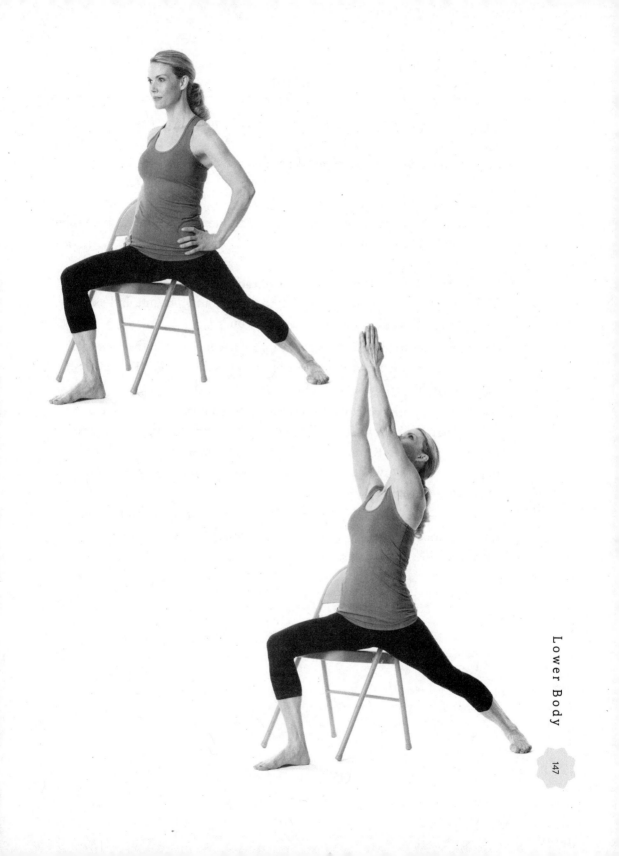

147

Warrior II

Virabhadrasana II is the stance the soldier took to set his aim on his prize. The torso stays even between the hips in this pose to remind us not to rush into battle or hang too far back. A true warrior can stand in his center and act when he's ready.

Works Your: Legs, buttocks, hips, abs, and arms

Try This: When you want to focus, need some confidence, or want to strengthen your lower half and feel strong and stable

1. Start seated with your butt at the edge of the chair and toward the middle of the seat, so you can pivot to the left to sit on your right side and extend your left leg off the chair and back behind you.

2. Open your hips to the left side so your right knee is bent and the back leg is straight. Let your left foot angle out slightly more than in warrior I, but still keep the ankle farther back than the toes.

3. Make sure you feel your feet grounded on the floor, and use your outer hips to keep the bent knee tracking forward and not rolling inward or off the chair. Press firmly through the back leg and outer foot and feel the lift in the inner left thigh. Keep your hips even in the chair and your torso directly above them.

4. Stretch your arms out to the sides and look over your right hand and hold for 5 to 8 breaths. Come back to center and perform on the left side. Repeat each side 2 to 3 more times.

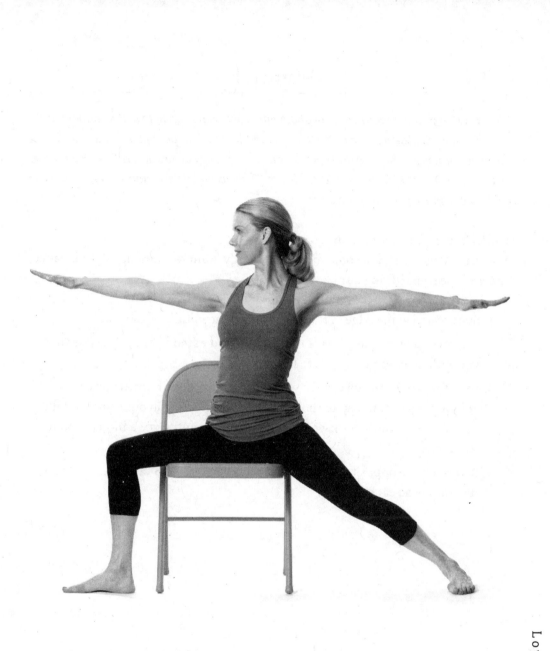

Warrior III

Warrior III in a chair requires a lot of abdominal control and strength in the buttocks. It's a super fun and challenging one to try, though, and it's the final pose in the virabhadrasana series. According to lore, the soldier finally launches off and catches his princess in this pose. When you are feeling like you could really use the focus and determination to go after your goals and dreams, give this pose a try.

Works Your: Buttocks, core, and back

Try This: When you want some focus and energy, want to challenge your balance, or could use some lift in your backside

1. Start seated at the edge of the chair toward the middle of the seat.

2. Inch over toward the left side of the chair and extend your left leg behind you with the toes pressing into the floor.

3. Lean forward until you can lift your back leg up off the floor. If you can't lift your leg, try to come up to the tips of your toes. Stretch your arms straight back or out to the sides if you feel steady and want to try a more difficult variation.

4. Repeat on the opposite side, holding each side for 5 to 8 breaths. Try 2 to 3 repetitions on each leg.

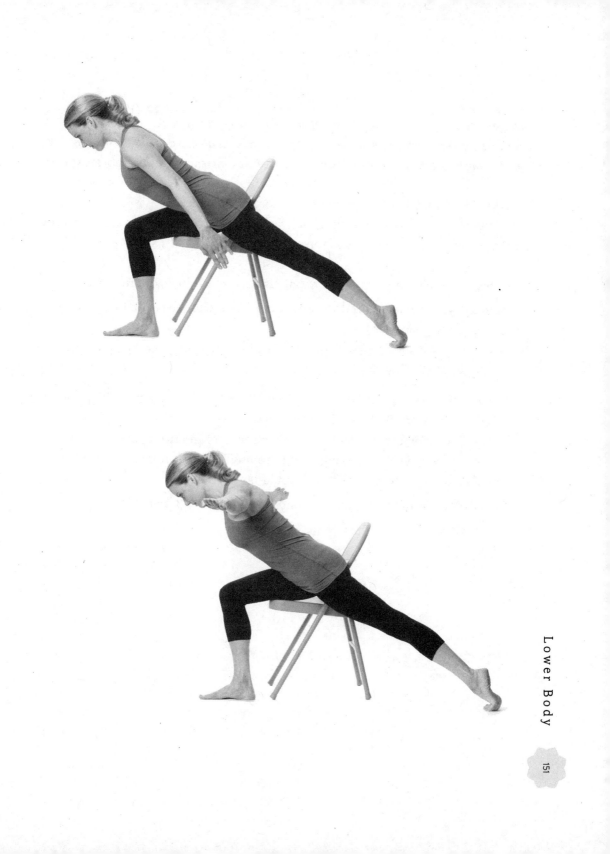

Lunge

Lunges are awesome for building strength in the thighs and buttocks. Lunging in a chair can also help lengthen the quadriceps and psoas muscles almost better than standing. Try alternating between the lunge and warrior I to see the difference in the angle of the stretch.

Works Your: Hips, quads, hamstrings, buttocks, and core
Try This: When your legs and lower back feel stiff, when you need a good release, or when you want to strengthen and tone your thighs

1. Start seated at the edge of your chair and inch your hips toward the left.

2. Reach your left leg behind you and press the toes into the floor. Keep squaring your hips forward.

3. Really press through your right foot and your left leg. Feel the incredible stretch in the front of the left thigh.

4. Keep your hands on your hips, or lift them up to the ceiling with the palms facing inward and shoulder-width apart.

5. For a variation that stretches open the shoulders and front body and gives you an even deeper opening in the front of the back thigh, arch up and back, coming into more of a crescent lunge pose.

6. Hold for 8 to 10 breaths on each side, and repeat 2 to 3 more times.

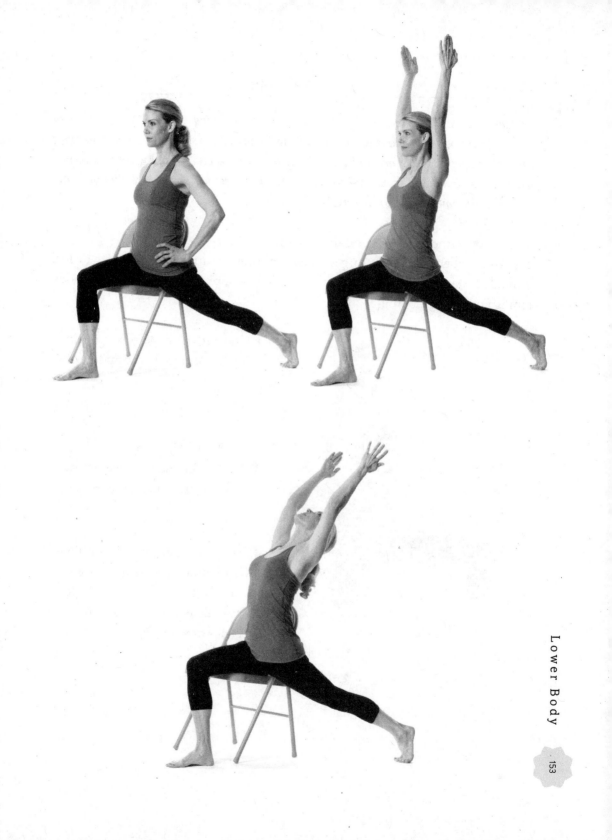

Goddess Squat

Goddess squats and squats in general are helpful for opening up the hips and building strength in the buttocks and legs. The great thing about doing a squat in a chair is the extra support you get. Many of my students can't keep their heels on the floor when they go into a deep squat. Squats bring blood flow to the pelvic floor region (thus are great for pregnant women and women trying to conceive).

Works Your: Abdominals, core, and inner thighs

Try This: When you want to get some feminine creative energy, need to feel grounded, want to connect with mother earth, or are craving some lower body toning and strengthening

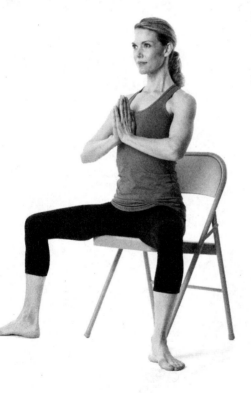

1. Start at the edge of your seat with your hips in the middle of the chair.

2. Open each leg out to its own side as wide as you can and turn the toes out at an angle.

3. Press your hands together at your heart center in a prayer shape and hold for 8 to 10 breaths.

4. For more advanced toning, try lifting your seat up a few inches from the chair. Hold as long as you can, then lower back down. Repeat 3 to 5 times.

Hamstrings

Stretching our hamstrings helps us maintain better posture and reduces stress felt in the lower back. The following options progressively increase in intensity, so play around with them and always remember it's okay to bend your knees. Each time someone tells me, "I can't touch my toes," I say, "Of course you can, you just need to bend your knees!" The most important thing to remember when forward bending is that our hips and buttocks are part of our back. When practicing these exercises, create an origami fold from the base of your sitz bones.

Straight Back Fold • Forward Fold

Leg on Ledge Fold • Advanced Hamstring Stretch

Straight Back Fold

Learning to hinge forward while maintaining a straight back requires a lot of focus and the proper muscular energy. Straight back fold teaches us to engage our core muscles to initiate a forward bend. This is personally one of my favorite stretches for the lower back. You can feel the entire lower back region lengthening as you open up your hamstrings. For those who suffer from herniated discs that are bulging out, this is a safe forward bend.

Works Your: Abdominals, lower back, and hamstrings
Try This: To feel a deep release in your hamstrings and lower back, to improve your flexibility, or to engage your core

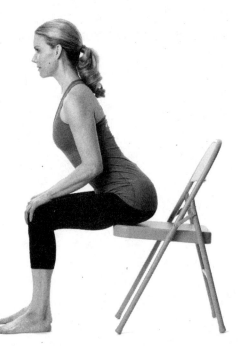

1. Start seated at the middle to front edge of the chair with both feet firmly planted on the floor.

2. Lean forward, keeping the back as flat as possible.

3. Concentrate on lifting your abdominals in and up and opening your chest. Hinge from the hips and continue going forward until you feel a gentle stretch in your hamstrings and lower back.

4. Hold for 5 to 8 breaths.

Our hamstrings can often feel very intense, so it's smart to take it slowly, and in a chair you can really modify the exercise and go at your own pace.

Forward Fold

Forward bends are great for decompressing the spine and mind. Whenever you want to really let go or need some brain drain, take a forward fold. You will notice immediately the amount of tension you carry in your back when you release over your legs. It may be uncomfortable at first, but use deep breaths to relax.

Works Your: Lower back and hamstrings
Try This: For relief in the backs of the thighs or to feel refreshed and enlightened

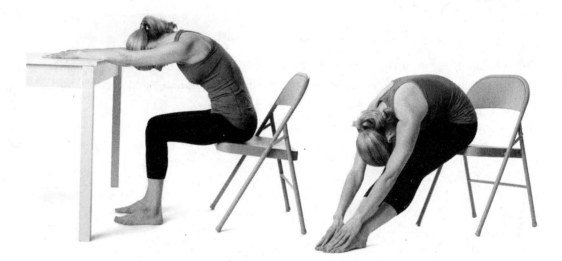

1. From the same starting position as your straight back fold, fold forward, letting your back round. If you have a desk or table in front of you, you can place your elbows and forehead on it.

2. For a deeper, full-body stretch, straighten your legs and fold all the way over until your hands are by your feet and your upper body is hanging like a rag doll.

3. You will feel a stretch and release in the back, particularly the lower back, and hamstrings. Hold for 8 to 10 breaths.

Leg on Ledge Fold

If you have a desk, a table, or another chair in front of you, you can practice a deeper seated hamstring stretch by placing one leg out in front of you on the prop. (I'm a crazy yogi and actually do this on the seat in front of me in the airplane with my leg up high—before the person sitting in front of me boards.)

Works Your: Hamstrings, lower back, and lower abdominals
Try This: When you need to stretch the backs of the legs, if you suffer from deep vein thrombosis, or if you are an active athlete and, once deskbound, find your muscles cramping up

1. Start seated at the edge of the chair.
2. Lengthen your right leg out in front of you and place the heel on the chair, table, or desk. Make sure to engage the quadriceps. Lengthen forward and over the straight extended leg.
3. Hold for 5 to 8 breaths and repeat on the opposite side.

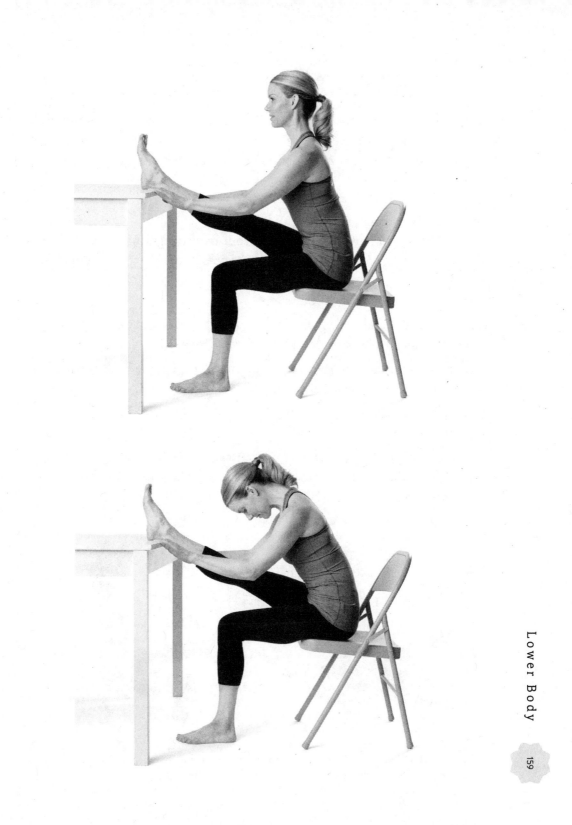

Advanced Hamstring Stretch

I couldn't live without this stretch. It not only opens up the entire back, side, and inner thighs, but it also works the core and releases the lower back. It's one of the exercises I do almost every day. For this stretch you can also use a strap, belt, or towel if you can't hold your foot or ankle.

Works Your: Hamstrings, arms, abs, and legs
Try This: When you really want to stretch your hamstrings, inner thighs, and IT band (a band of fascial tissue that runs from the outside of the leg to the upper shin)

1. Start seated at the edge of your chair.

2. Sitting up nice and tall, take hold of your right ankle and extend your leg straight out in front of you. Hold here for five breaths.

3. Next, try bringing the leg closer to your face, keeping the back as straight as possible. Hold for another five breaths.

4. Sit up tall again and try opening the leg to the right side for another five breaths.

5. Finally bring the leg across the midsection and to the left for a hamstring and IT stretch. Hold for five more breaths, release the leg, and repeat on the left side.

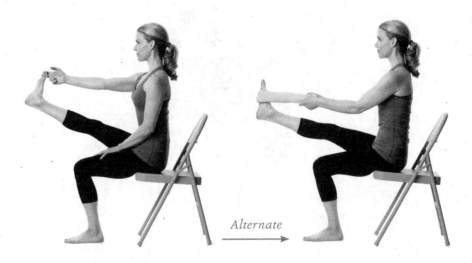

Alternate

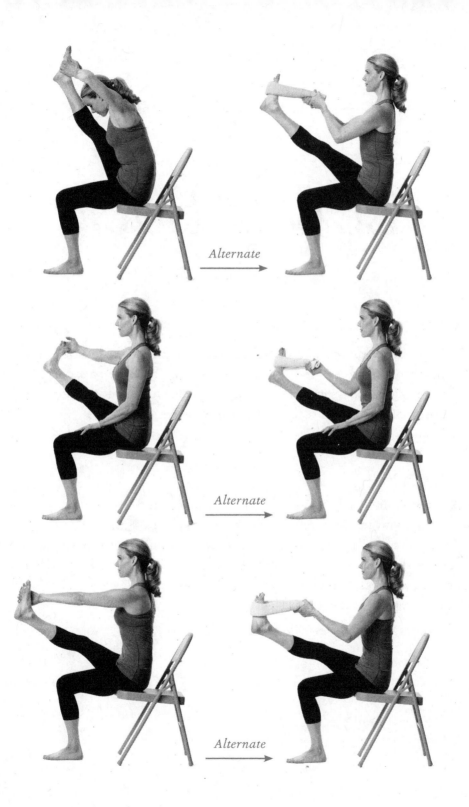

Alternate

Alternate

Alternate

8

Lower Back

Once you've warmed up by opening up and strengthening your legs, it's easier to open up and release your lower back. The lower back can feel quite fragile, and it's important to stay connected to the breath and really use the abdominals to support each one of these exercises.

Oh, my aching back! I can't tell you how many students and people I come across in my teaching and life who have back issues. Sitting for prolonged periods of time can definitely lead to and/or exacerbate back issues. When we sit, our hip flexors shorten in front and pull on our lower back. Also, many of us slouch in our chairs, which can lead to compressed discs over time. Tight hips, hamstrings, and quadriceps all lead to low back pain.

Back pain is one of the most debilitating symptoms to have, and sitting can really exacerbate it. It's crucial if you suffer from low back pain to do these moves to help ease the discomfort. Strengthening and stretching the legs, hips, and lower back (along with the core work you've already been introduced to) can make a world of difference in the health of your back and spine. Having more open hips and hamstrings will surely help release the back as well.

Sherman et al. (doi:10.1001/archinternmed.2001.524) published a randomized study of 228 adults with chronic back pain to determine whether yoga is more effective than conventional stretching or a self-care book. They concluded that yoga classes were more effective than a self-care book but not more effective than stretching classes in improving function and reducing symptoms of chronic low back pain, with benefits lasting several months. Yoga and stretching are particularly appealing because they are safe, inexpensive, and highly accessible to most people.

It's amazing to discover how much you can open up and release your back with a chair. Most of us stay parked in one position for way too long and all of these exercises remind us to keep moving. When we are stagnant in our body, especially our lower half, our energy is like a muddy puddle that keeps getting more weighed down. Yoga helps us clear the waters and stay clean and healthy.

Stretch and Strengthen Your Back Muscles

The following collection of exercises can be done in any order, but it's nice to start with a gentle backbend to warm up. Make sure to really tap into your ujjayi breathing since it calms the nervous system. Also remember to sit tall at the edge of your seat with your feet planted firmly on the floor.

Backbend Arch

For a simple lower back opener you can begin with a gentle backbend on the chair. I often like to close my eyes in this posture and visualize the release in the back while using my core to stabilize and support the stretch.

Works Your: Lower and upper back

Try This: Whenever you need some fresh oxygen in the body, feel your lower back tensing or tightening up, or feel your energy or mood lagging

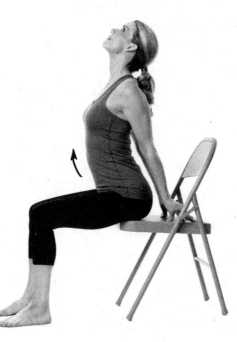

1. Start seated at the edge of your chair and place your hands behind you with the fingers facing away from the hips.

2. Prop yourself up on your fingertips and draw your sacrum region in and upward to lift your lower back.

3. Follow the backbend all the way up the chest to the shoulder blades and open up the entire front body. Hold and breathe for 8 to 10 breaths.

Cat/Cow

I've already introduced you to cat/cow pose in the "Warm-ups" chapter of this book. It is covered here again because of its therapeutic relief for the back. Cat/cow is truly like giving yourself a massage.

Works Your: Upper and lower back and abdominals
Try This: After you've done your roll downs (page 166) or as another way to release the spine and open up the back

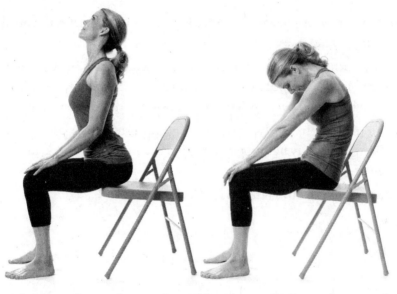

1. Sit at the edge of your chair with your feet flat on the floor. Place your hands on your knees and inhale, lifting your chest and sticking your hips out behind you. It's as if you're doing the pelvic arch forward but lifting the arch all the way up into your entire back.

2. Lift your gaze, open your chest, and gently squeeze your shoulder blades together.

3. On your exhalation, round your chest, scoop in your belly, and curl under your tailbone as you drop your head toward your sternum (like a Halloween cat).

4. Repeat for a series of ten cycles.

Roll Downs

Roll downs are like a wave in the spine, creating space in the vertebrae and opening up the back. They can be done as a morning warm-up or any time you want to release the kinks in your spine.

Works Your: Spine, back, and abdominals

Try This: When you need some more freedom in your spine, to release your back, or to get more creative flow in your day

1. Start seated with your feet on the floor hip-width apart and your hands hanging at your sides.

2. From your head, start rounding down through the spine. Use an exhalation and let the forehead release forward and the weight of the head continue to bring you over until the top of your head is by your thighs.

3. On an inhalation, slowly start stacking the vertebrae as you round up to sit. Draw your belly button to your spine to protect your back, and feel the articulation as you round up.

4. Continue rolling down and up for 5 to 8 cycles.

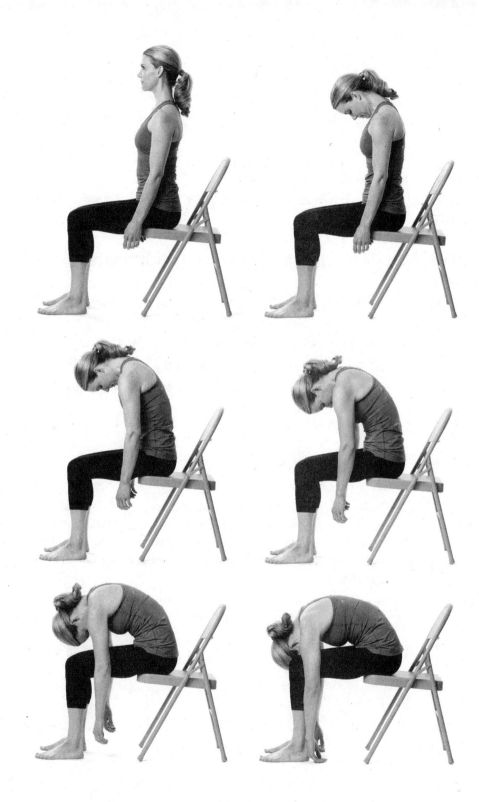

Lower Back Circles

For this next exercise, imagine stirring a pot and freeing up your lower back by circling around.

Works Your: Lower back and abdominals

Try This: When you need to release your lower back, want to stir some things up, or need some creative energy

1. Start seated with your feet hip-width apart and your hands resting on your knees.

2. Inhale and start to circle your torso around in a clockwise rotation, making sure to initiate the movement from the base of the spine. Circle 8 to 10 times in this direction, then stop and start to spin the other way.

3. Let the movement free up your entire spine and body. Have fun and let go. Continue circling in one direction and then the other for 2 to 3 minutes.

In life we can sometimes get stuck in our own way. I feel like this exercise helps us get unstuck on a mental level and see the whole perspective. So much of life is forward movement, and when we spin our torsos in this way, it really helps keep our bodies safe and functional and our energy circulating.

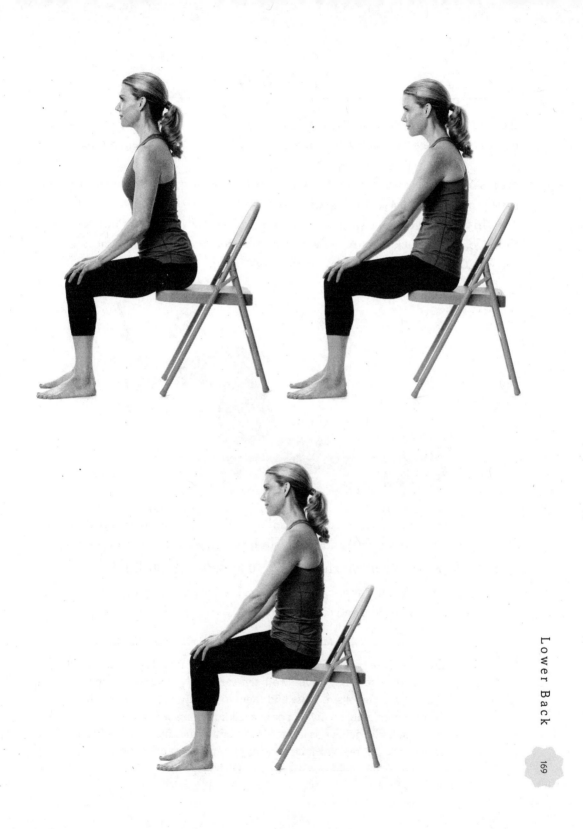

Back Relief

This posture is one of the most therapeutic back releases. Back relief is a simple inversion and great for relieving tension in the lower back and letting the blood flow in reverse.

Works Your: This exercise is mainly restorative and soothes the central nervous system as well as releases the legs and back.

Try This: When you have the space in your office to close the door and let everything go, if your back is aching, if your legs are tired, or if you're at home and need some TLC (you can also do this with your legs on the couch)

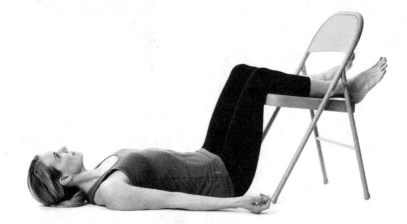

1. Lie down on your back (prop yourself up with pillows or a folded blanket if you want more support) and edge your hips in toward the base of the chair.

2. Place your legs up on the chair with your knees bent at 90 degrees.

3. Hold here for as long as you would like to, then gently take your legs off the chair, roll to one side, and come up to sit.

Inversions are great for the lymphatic system and for letting the blood flow in reverse. They have also been said to be good for the thyroid gland and metabolism. I just find them to be super relaxing and much needed after being on my feet or in a chair for long periods of time. You might look silly doing this in the airport or at your office, but the beauty of this pose is it really can be done anywhere and at any time!

Backbend

The antidepressants of yoga, backbends are great for opening up the chest region and getting more oxygen into the lungs. Back bending reverses all the forward bending and rounded shoulder posturing that we do throughout the day. Backbends are also great for strengthening the hips, buttocks, and hamstrings.

Works Your: Lower and upper back

Try This: When you want some mood-boosting energy, feel overwhelmed or frustrated, or want to strengthen and tone your backside

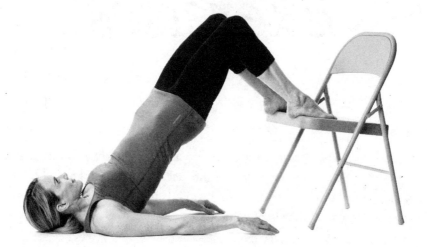

1. Start lying on your back with your knees bent and legs resting on the seat of the chair.

2. Press your feet into the chair or the edge of the seat (make sure the chair is sturdy enough and will stay put when you push into it) and start to lift your hips up off the floor.

3. Press your hands into the floor and puff your chest to your chin to really stretch open the front body.

4. Draw your belly button to your spine and engage your hamstrings as you lengthen your tailbone and lower back area.

5. Hold for 5 to 8 breaths and then lower down. Repeat 3 to 4 times.

9

Standing Exercises

The best thing you can do throughout the day is to get off your butt! Set a timer on your computer or phone for the last five minutes of each hour to remind you it's time to stand up. And while you're at it, try some of these standing poses with the aid of your chair.

There's research that says if you can reduce the amount of sitting to less than three hours a day, you can increase your life expectancy by two years! Let's get moving!

Walk to the watercooler to refill your water bottle, use the stairs instead of the elevator, go to a colleague's desk instead of calling, make sure to get outside and take a walk for lunch, or stand up to do some yoga using a chair. It's awesome to have a chair to use for a prop; it allows us to do certain standing yoga postures with more ease and control. I certainly found this to be true while pregnant.

There are times when you can get so engaged with your work on the computer or a program on Netflix that before you know it, you've been on your seat for too long. But humans are designed to move and not stay stuck in one position for extended periods of time. The repercussions from sitting all day long are worse than we realize. The most interesting thing about the studies done on prolonged hours of sitting is that one hour of exercise doesn't offset all the risk factors. The goal with these exercises is that they become built-in moments throughout your day to get up and get moving, which will help you be at ease and find a comfort level in your body that will make you happier, healthier, and live longer!

I find we limit ourselves with excuses for why we can't move, when the reality is it's easier than we think. I've found myself at the airport doing hamstring stretches on a chair, or at the doctor's office and using the waiting room chair for a downward-facing dog. I rarely get odd looks; I usually have people asking me how they can join in!

Get Off Your Butt!

Now that you're energized, get ready to try some standing yoga moves with the aid of a chair. Be creative and have fun. You'll need a little more space for these, so make sure your area is open. Feel free to practice in shoes or, if you can and want to, take off your shoes and socks—you may find you have better balance through your feet.

Quad Stretch

Our quads and hip flexors get overly tight and shortened when we sit for hours at a time. Tight hip flexors pull on the lower back and set us up for pain in the back and compression in the organs. When our psoas is shortened and weak, it can mess with our digestive, reproductive, and other internal organs.

Works Your: Front leg muscles, particularly the quadriceps, and hip flexors
Try This: When you feel stress boiling up, want to give the entire front body a stretch, or want to combat slouching

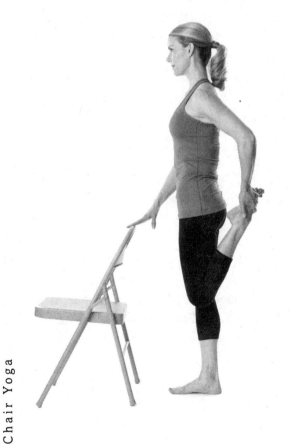

1. Stand behind your desk chair and place your right hand on the back for balance.

2. Reach your left hand back to grab the front of your left foot and gently draw the heel in toward the buttocks.

3. Lengthen your left knee toward the floor, tuck your tailbone under, and lift your chest. Hold for 5 to 8 breaths before switching sides.

Figure 4

Our outer thighs and external rotators play a similar role as the quadriceps and hip flexors when it comes to the lower back. If our outer hips are tight, our back suffers as well. Many people develop sciatica or piriformis syndrome over time when their hips are overly tight or weak. It's crucial to keep the entire hip region open and strong.

Works Your: Outer hips, inner thighs, buttocks, and abs
Try This: Whenever you have dead butt syndrome, have discomfort in the hips or back, or need to get rid of junk or stale energy in the trunk

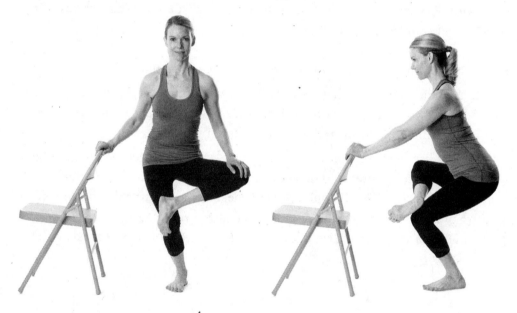

1. Start standing next to your chair and place your right hand on the back for support.

2. Cross your left ankle over your right knee, turning the left knee open to the side.

3. Start to bend the right leg and lower down as far as comfortable until you feel a stretch in the outer left hip and buttocks. Hold for 8 to 10 breaths, stand up, and switch sides.

4. If you need more support for balance, face the back of the chair and hold on with both hands.

Lunge

Tone the buttocks and thighs with these lunges. Lunges give us strength and help us find the energy to support ourselves with our legs. Lunges are great for the quadriceps, hamstrings, glutes, and abdominals. This standing lunge is a good way to begin to get a sense of where the weight should be on the front foot as well as to feel a good stretch in the front side of the back leg.

Works Your: Hips (especially the hip flexors), buttocks, quadriceps, calves, and hamstrings

Try This: For pain or compression in the lower back, to tone your buttocks, or to stretch out your legs

1. Stand facing your chair and place your right foot on the seat.

2. Hold the back of the chair as you lean forward into the lunge to stretch the front of your left hip flexors and quadriceps. Make sure to draw your lower abdominals in and up and keep your chest lifted.

3. Press firmly into the front foot and don't let the knee get too far past the front ankle. You want to make sure you don't put any stress on the knee joint, which can lead to injury over time. For added difficulty, bring your hands to your front thigh or raise them above you. Engage your buttocks and hamstrings on the right leg and hold for 8 to 10 breaths. Repeat on the opposite leg.

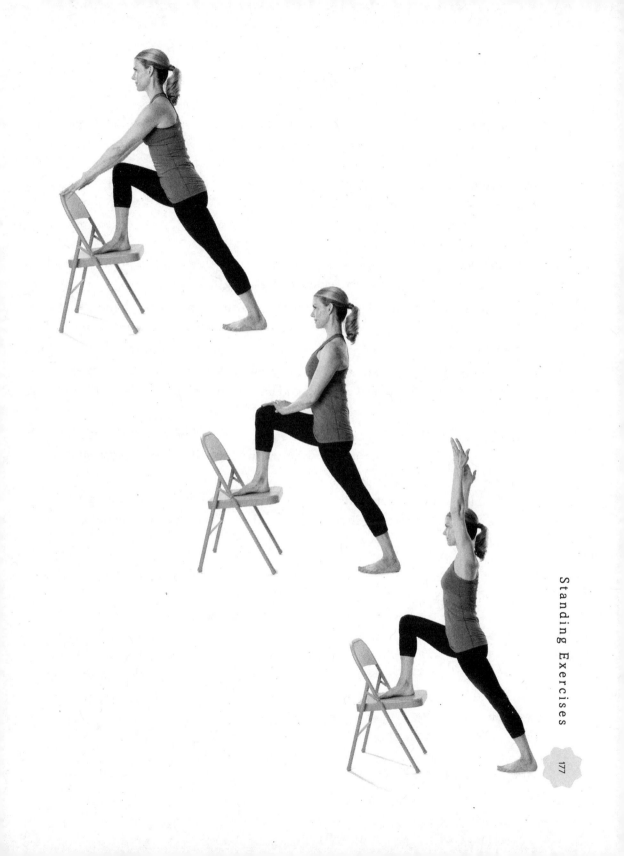

High Lunge

For a deeper stretch and a more challenging strengthening pose, you can practice lunging standing beside your chair and using the chair for support.

Works Your: Quads, hips, hamstrings, and glutes
Try This: When you want a full-body pose, need to get the blood flowing, or want to boost your metabolic rate

1. Stand tall sideways behind your chair. Hold on to the chairback with your right hand and step your left leg back a leg's length.

2. Lunge the right knee deeply until the thigh is almost parallel with the seat of the chair. Make sure to keep the knee above the ankle to protect your knee.

3. Press firmly through your left heel and lengthen behind your left knee. Engage your right gluteal muscles and anchor the entire right foot to the floor.

4. Make sure to deeply engage your abdominals and hold for 8 to 10 breaths. Stand up and switch to the other side, or turn around to face the opposite direction to work the other side.

5. As you get comfortable with the pose, work on extending your arms up to the ceiling, palms facing in toward each other, or just place your hands on your hips.

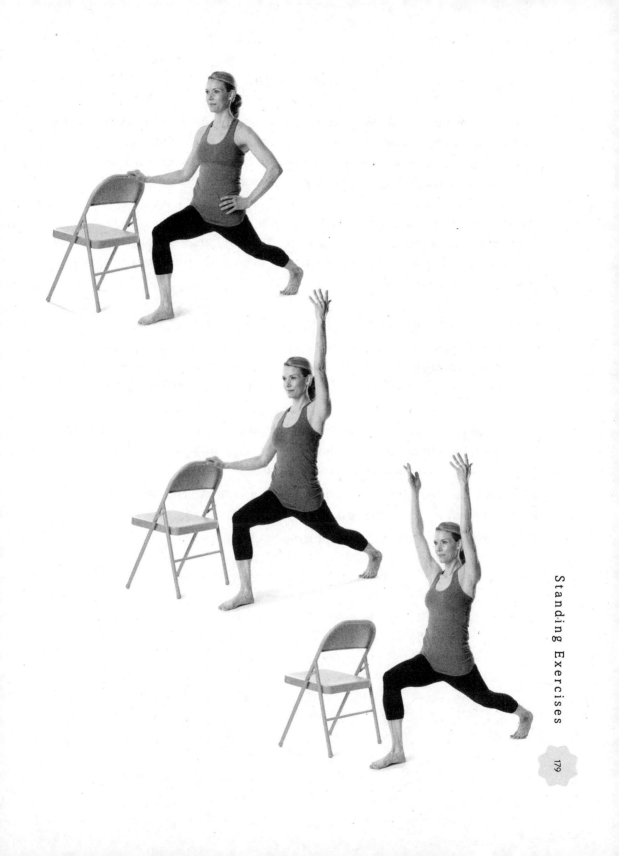

Low Lunge

Low lunge stretches the front of the back leg deeper than high lunge and really opens up the entire psoas, hip flexor, and quadriceps region. Low lunge is also a little bit more passive than high lunge since the back knee is dropped. You may want a towel or extra padding under the knee if you find this pose uncomfortable on the top of the knee.

Works Your: Hip flexors, quadriceps, hamstrings, and glutes

Try This: For relief in the front of the legs, to release fight-or-flight tension, if you are sore from a big workout, when you want to open up the front body and lungs, or you need some lower back relief

1. Stand tall beside your chair. Hold on to the chairback and step your left leg back a leg's length.

2. Lunge the right knee deeply until the thigh is almost parallel with the seat of the chair. Always keep the knee above your ankle to prevent stress on the knee.

3. Drop your left knee to the floor and release the top of the foot along the floor. Press firmly into the front leg as you let your hips release forward to stretch the left hip flexors, quad, and psoas.

4. Keep the abdominals engaged as well as the buttocks. For a more advanced variation, try to lift one or both arms above your head.

5. Hold for 5 to 8 breaths and repeat on the opposite side.

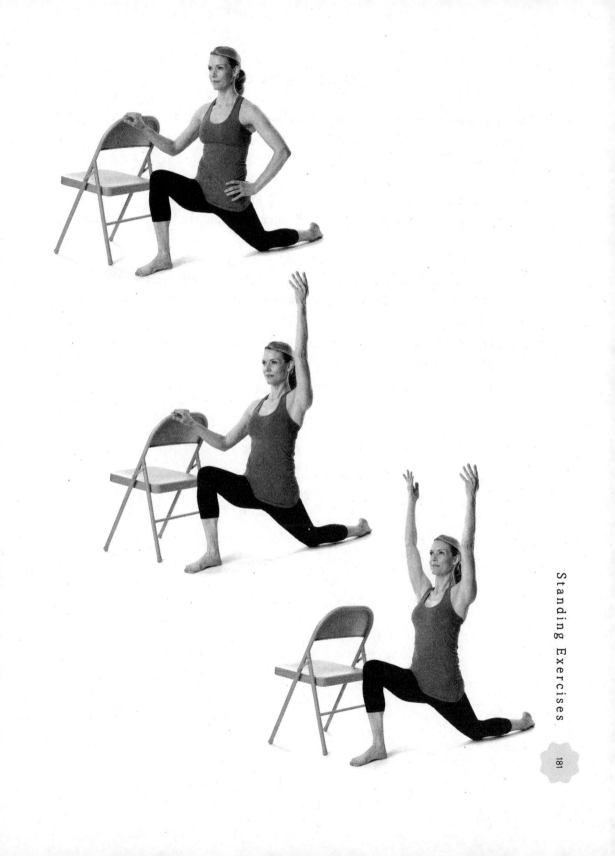

Hamstring Stretch

There are many ways to stretch the hamstrings, and each exercise hits the legs in a slightly different way. This particular hamstring stretch I feel through the entire back of my leg, even my calves.

Works Your: Legs (especially the hamstrings), lower back, and abs
Try This: For an achy or stiff back, or a deeper stretch in the backs of the legs and the calf muscles

1. Stand facing your chair and place your right heel on the seat of the chair (for a more advanced variation, you can even place your heel up on the chairback).
2. Engage the front of your thigh and hinge forward over your leg until you feel a deep stretch in the back of the leg.
3. Hold for 5 to 8 breaths and then switch legs.

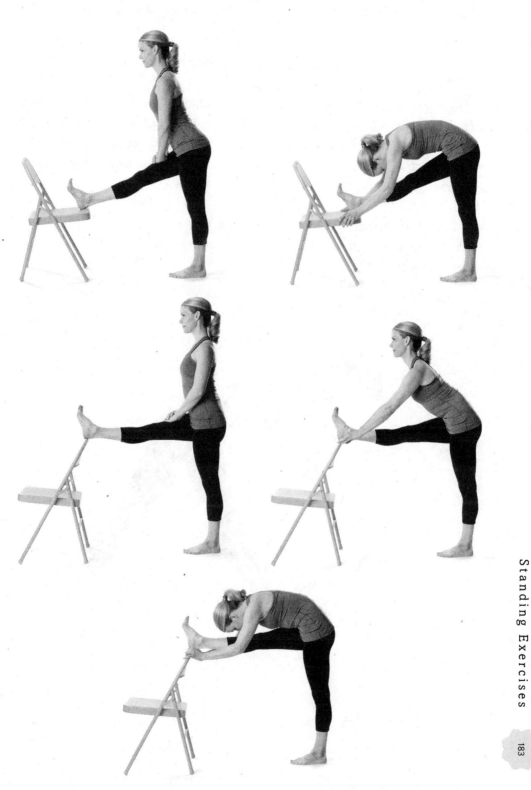

Intense Side Stretch

To get the backs of the hamstrings open, it's important to stretch them daily and to use props that can assist you. When we keep our hamstrings loose and flexible, we can release the pull and strain on our back. Although we are primarily lengthening the backs of the thighs, we are also working on stretching the sides of the waist and lengthening the spine over the front thigh.

Works Your: Hamstrings, quadriceps, back, and abs

Try This: For extra length in the backs of your thighs or when you feel achy in the lower back and body

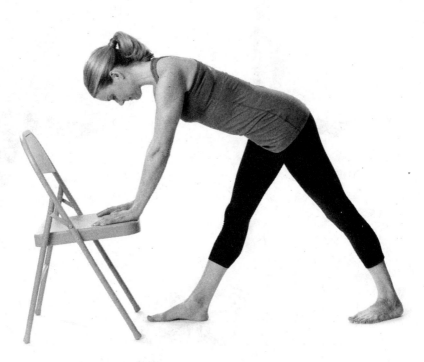

1. Stand facing your chair with your right foot forward and your left foot about half a leg's length behind you.

2. Press the outer edge of the left foot into the floor and hinge forward at your waist, placing your hands on the seat of the chair.

3. Try to keep your back nice and long at first and both legs straight. Engage the quadriceps muscles and the area above the kneecaps.

4. After 5 to 8 breaths with the back flat, lay your chest over your front thigh for an even deeper stretch and hold for 5 to 8 more breaths. Repeat on the opposite side. You can also do this exercise standing beside the chair and placing one hand on the chair as you fold forward.

Pigeon on Chair

Our outer hips and external rotators can really get tight after sitting for hours on end. It's important to listen to your knees if you have knee issues or feel any extra strain in them when you try pigeon. If so, you can always go back to figure 4 (page 175) or ankle to knee (page 140) to get a similar stretch in the outer hips.

Works Your: Outer hips, inner thighs, hamstrings, glutes, and abs
Try This: When you want to stretch out your seat, need to relieve sciatic or hip pain, feel tightness in your back, or want an advanced deep hip opener

1. Stand facing the side of the chair. Place your outer right calf on the seat of the chair with the knee toward the outside of the right hip and the foot as parallel to the chair's edge as possible (listen to your body and don't push too far).
2. Gently inch your left leg back until you get settled onto the outer upper hip and feel an incredible hip opening. Hold for 5 to 8 breaths and gently come back up to stand. Repeat on the left side.

Variation:

1. Place your outer calf on the upper edge of the chairback (this works great in airport chairs) and stand tall or hinge forward for an extremely deep hip opener and great balance challenge.
2. Keep your abdominals engaged and hold for 5 to 8 breaths, then switch legs.

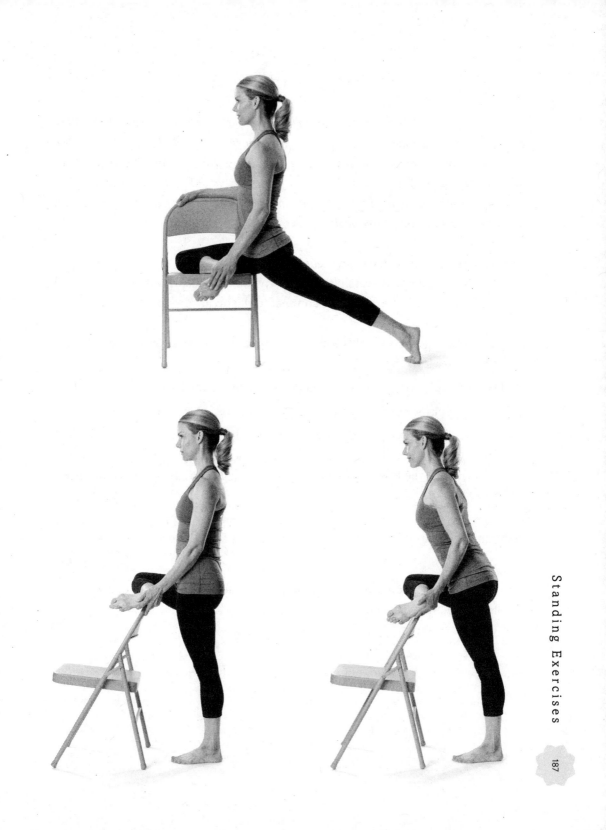

Downward-Facing Dog

This is one of the best yoga poses for strengthening and stretching the entire body. When using the chair to perform downward dog, you can really stretch the upper body easily since you're not putting all of your weight on your arms. You can also find length in your back as you imagine your hips moving away from your shoulders. Lastly, you won't have to worry much about tight hamstrings as in this variation and can bend the knees slightly to feel the hips tilt up and move back.

Works Your: Arms, abs, back, and legs

Try This: For a full-body stretch; to release the upper back, shoulders, head, neck, and legs; or to refresh the mind and connect to the breath

1. Stand facing the back of the chair and place your hands on the chairback shoulder-width apart.
2. Walk your feet back until your chest is parallel to the floor.
3. Engage your lower abdominals and lift your ribs up away from the floor.
4. Think of arching out of the lower back and lifting your hips up and away from your shoulders. Bend your knees to help pull you back even more, then engage the kneecaps and lengthen the legs straight again. Hold for 8 to 10 breaths.

Variation:

1. Place the hands on the seat of the chair instead to create more of an angle from the hips to the head.
2. Hold for 8 to 10 breaths.

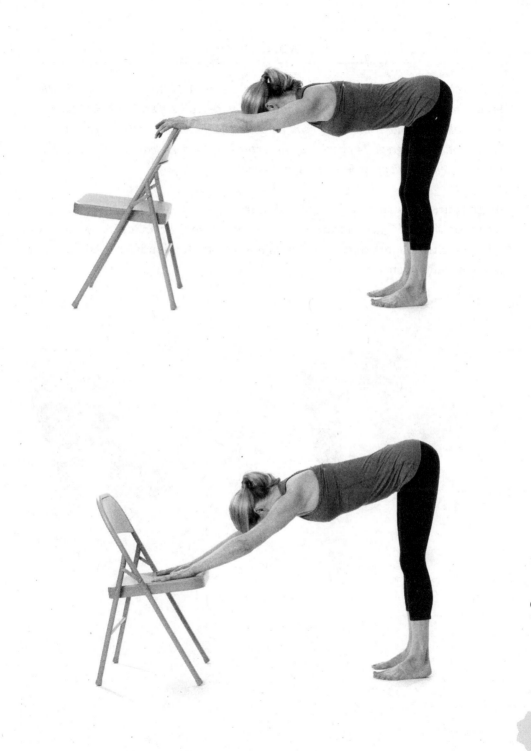

Forward Hang

Sometimes we just need to let go. Forward hangs are incredible for dropping it all. When I'm hanging forward, I love to imagine a little door at the crown of my head that I can open up to let all the mental trash in my head fall to the floor and just say bye-bye to forever. Forward hangs are great for opening up the entire back body, releasing tight hamstrings, and letting tension out of the head, neck, and shoulder region.

Works Your: Hamstrings, back, and abdominals

Try This: When you need to drop the contents in your brain, open up the back body, stretch the hamstrings and lower back, release tension in the shoulders, or get some renewed energy

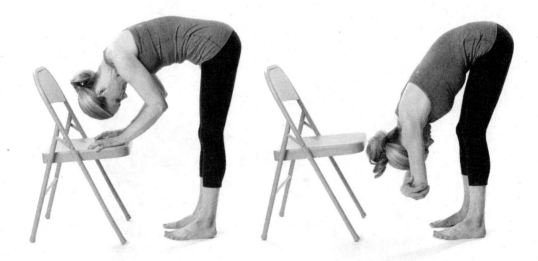

1. Stand facing your chair and put your hands on the seat of the chair as you slowly fold forward over your legs.

2. Go as far as you can and let your head hang heavy. Keep your hands on the chair for support or eventually let both hands hang toward the floor.

3. Make sure to keep the weight forward in the arches of the feet—don't sink back into the heels or lock the knees (bend the knees by all means if you need to)—and feel all the tension release out of your spine.

4. You can also hold opposite elbows and sway a little from side to side in your fold. Hold for 8 to 10 breaths before slowly rounding back up to stand, using the chair for support as much as you need to.

Standing Side Stretch

When you need a big release, any kind of side bend really helps to open up the lungs and waist for a deep breath of fresh air, as well as alleviating tension in the shoulders, waist, and lower back. Using a chair as a prop in a side stretch can help you go even deeper since you have the support and a tactile aid as you lengthen into the pose.

Works Your: Obliques, core, and arms

Try This: To relieve tension, when you need some deep breaths, or when you feel like you're shrinking from sitting too much.

1. Start standing with your right side next to the back of the chair.
2. Inhale and lift your left arm up alongside your ear and place your right hand on the top of the back of the chair. Exhale and lean to your right. Stay for 5 to 8 breaths, trying to keep the length in both sides as you stretch the entire left side. Make sure to press your shoulders down away from your ears. If you would like to, you can look up under the top arm to stretch the neck as well.
3. After your last deep exhalation, lift back up and turn around to repeat on the other side.

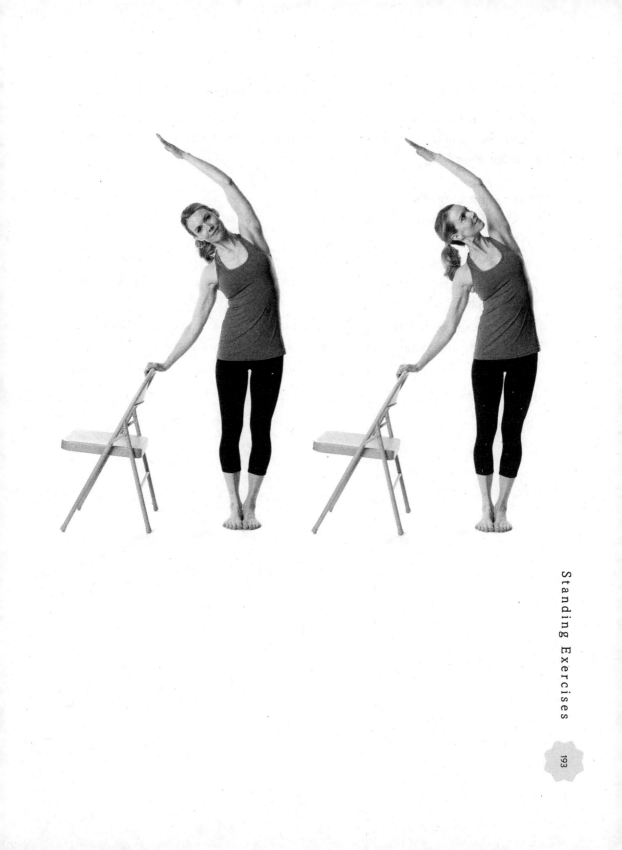

Standing Twist

Twists are great for digestion and spinal mobility. I love doing a twist midday when I need to reset things. I also like doing them after meals when I feel sluggish and need a little aid in moving things along.

Works Your: Core, obliques, legs, and arms
Try This: To stimulate digestion, refresh your mood, or get a new perspective

1. Start standing tall with your right side next to the back of your chair.
2. Place your right hand on the back of the chair and hug your right knee into your chest with your left hand.
3. Inhale a deep breath and take a twist to the right as you exhale. Continue inhaling and exhaling deeper into the twist for 5 to 8 breaths.
4. Repeat on the left side, by turning around and holding on to the chair with your left hand.

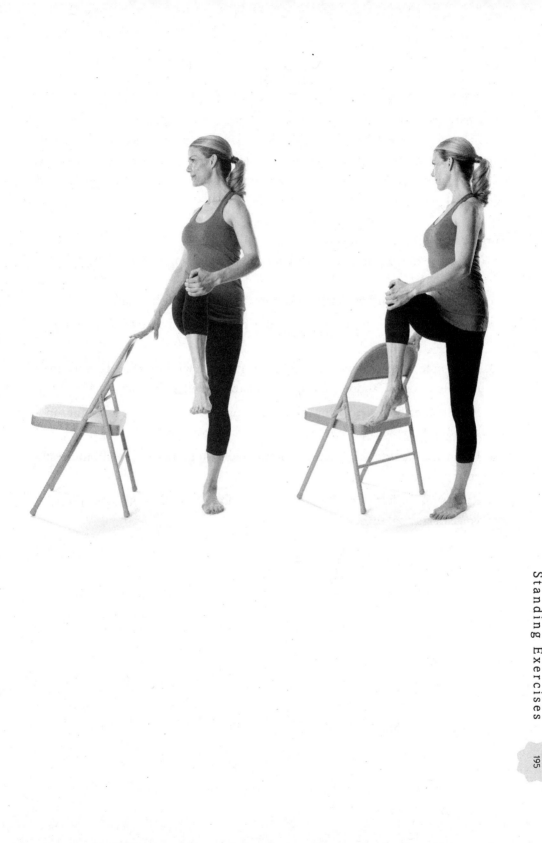

Tree

One of the classic yoga poses, tree is an incredible posture for helping us get grounded and to work on our balance. Whenever you feel like you're being pulled in too many directions, it's great to stop and stand in tree. Gather all of your energy back in and strengthen your foundation, spread your roots, and open your branches without letting the wind blow you over.

Works Your: Core, legs, arms, abs
Try This: To focus, get grounded, work on your balance, or tone your thighs

1. Start standing with your right side next to the back of the chair.
2. Take your left foot to the upper inner right thigh and turn the knee out to the side.
3. Hold on to the chair with the right hand to help with balance as you continue to draw the abdominals in and up and stabilize the core.
4. Press the left foot firmly into the right thigh without letting the right hip sink or fall to the right side. Stand tall and lift your chest.
5. When you feel steady, try pressing the palms together in prayer and test your balance.
6. Repeat on the left side. Hold on each side for 5 to 10 breaths or as long as you can stay balanced.

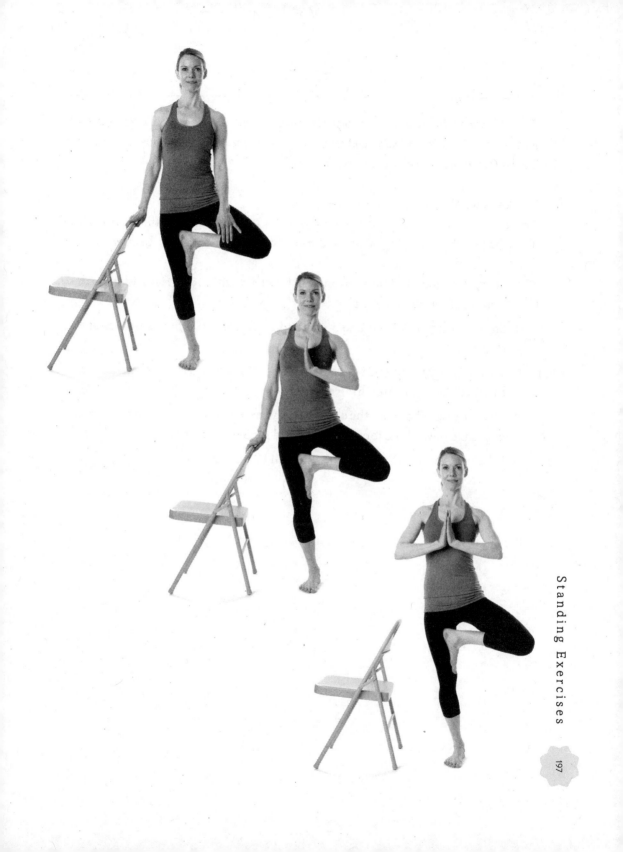

197

Triangle

The sides and waist are always important to stretch and open. One of the best poses in yoga for lengthening the torso and opening up the sides is triangle. Triangle pose also lengthens the inner thighs and tones the legs and abs.

Works Your: Waist, inner thighs, legs, and arms

Try This: When you need a pick-me-up, want to tone and lengthen through the sides, have tight inner thighs, or need some fresh air or a new perspective

1. Start standing slightly in front of the chair with your right foot in the middle of the chair's front legs.

2. Step your left foot back 2 to 3 feet and angle the left foot inward about 45 degrees.

3. Turn the right foot out 90 degrees. Lengthen your arms to the sides and hinge to the right, stretching as far as you can.

4. Place the right hand on the chair seat and extend the left arm up to the ceiling. Gaze toward the top hand and hold for 5 to 8 breaths.

5. Inhale to stand up and position yourself for the left side.

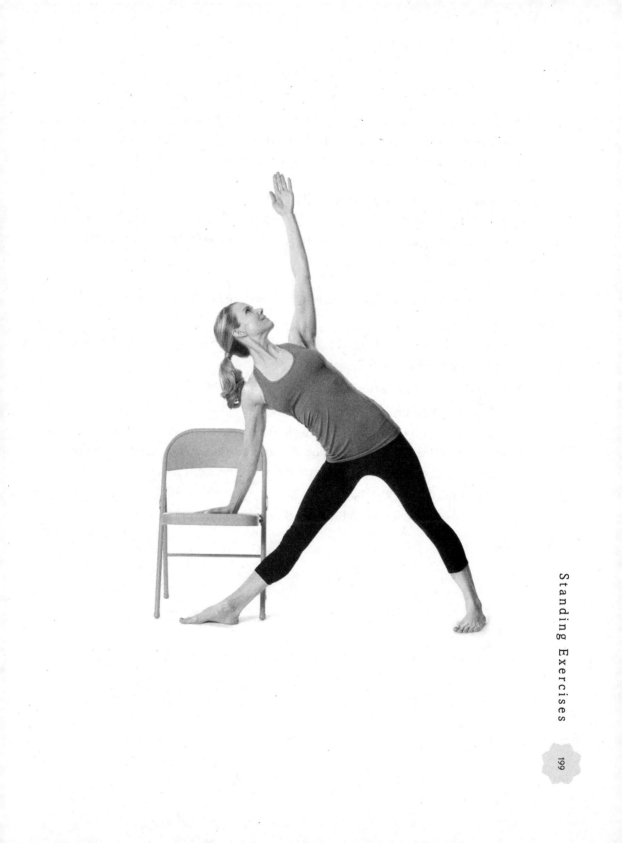

Standing Warrior I

Warrior poses are always some of the best yoga postures for strengthening the legs and helping to really build stamina in the body. When your energy is lagging, or when you need a mental and physical boost, get up out of your seat and strike a warrior pose.

Works Your: Legs, arms, and abdominals

Try This: To open up your front body; for tight hip flexors; when you need some confidence boosting or want to feel strong; or when you want to rev up your energy and metabolism

1. Start standing next to your chair and place your right hand on the chair-back.

2. Step your left foot back a full leg's length and turn the left foot so that it is angled forward at about 75 degrees.

3. Bend your right knee until the thigh is parallel with the floor without letting the knee go past the ankle.

4. Try to keep both hips forward facing and lift your arms up above your ears with the palms facing each other. For an additional challenge, press the palms together completely. To modify, keep the right hand on the chair and just lift the left arm up.

5. Hold and breathe for 5 to 8 breaths and repeat on the other side.

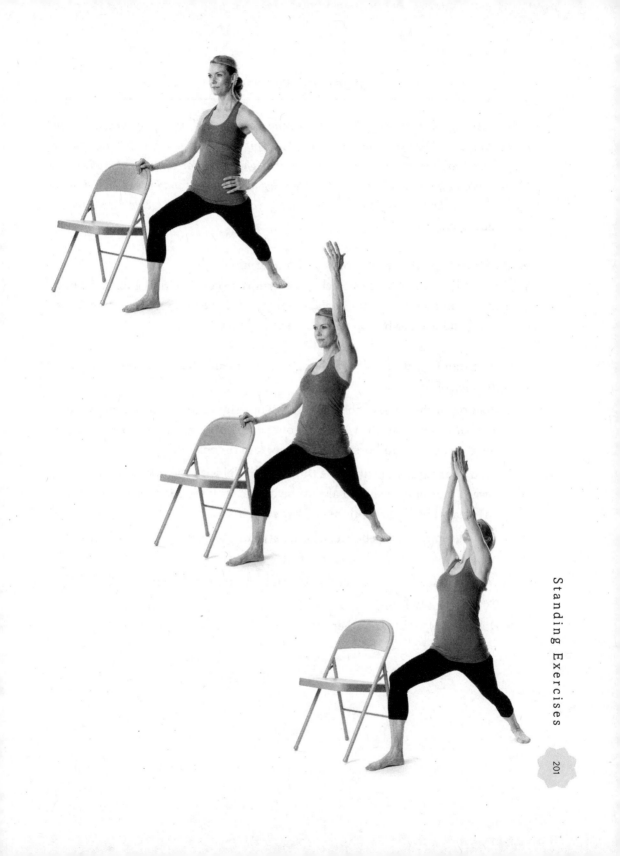

Standing Warrior II

Doing standing warriors with the aid of a chair helps to find proper alignment without having to strain. When you hold the back of the chair as you go into the postures, you can really steady yourself and make sure you have the right form. Warrior II is especially tricky for some people because of tight hips and weak leg muscles; the front knee often rolls in on itself. When you line yourself up with the chair leg, you can use it as a tactile aid to keep the knee tracking properly.

Works Your: Hips, thighs, buttocks, abs, and arms

Try This: When you want to stretch out the hips, need a burst of energy, want to tone and strengthen the glutes and abdominals, or have an extra important event or meeting and need to fire up your stamina and focus

1. Start standing at the back of the chair and line up your right foot with the front leg of the chair.

2. Hold on to the back of the chair with your right hand and step your left foot back a leg's length away from your right foot, angling the toes forward about 45 degrees and pressing the outer foot in the floor.

3. Bend your right knee until the thigh is parallel with the floor and guide it toward the chair (it should almost be in line with the seat). Make sure the knee stays above the ankle and doesn't roll in.

4. Try to keep your torso between both legs and draw your abdominals in and up.

5. When you feel steady, extend both arms out to the sides and gaze forward over your right fingers.

6. Hold for 8 to 10 breaths, then stand up and repeat on the left side.

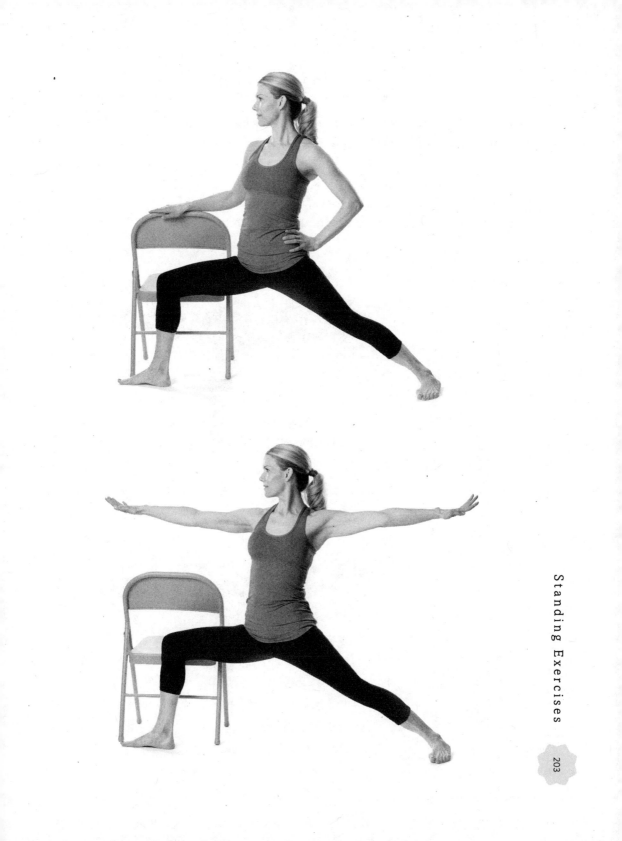

Standing Warrior III

To build focus; increase stamina and strength in the legs, core, and back; and boost your metabolism, warrior III is the best pose.

Works Your: Buttocks, legs, feet, back, and core
Try This: When you need some focus, lack confidence, need a boost of energy, or want to build your backside or tone and strengthen the legs

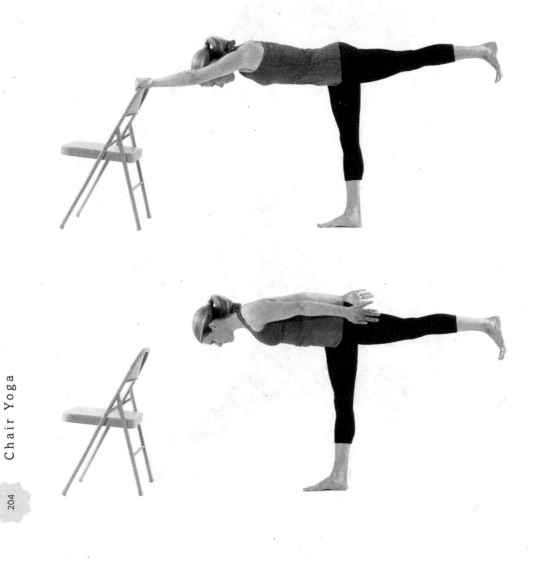

1. Start by standing at the back of your chair. Place your hands on the top of the chair back and walk backward until your upper body is parallel to the floor.

2. Lift your left leg up behind you with the toes pointing down to the floor. Try to level your hips (imagine you're balancing a teacup on your lower back).

3. You should form a stick from heel to head. When you feel comfortable you can try to let go of the chair and send your arms along your sides to test your balance.

4. Hold for 5 to 8 breaths on each side.

Butt Lifts

Sometimes we all just want a little quick toning for our backside. I threw this exercise in because it's fun and effective. Standing and doing butt lifts with the chair is challenging for the hips and buttocks and really gives you a nice lift in your rear.

Works Your: Buttocks, legs, back, and core
Try This: When you feel like breaking out your inner Jane Fonda

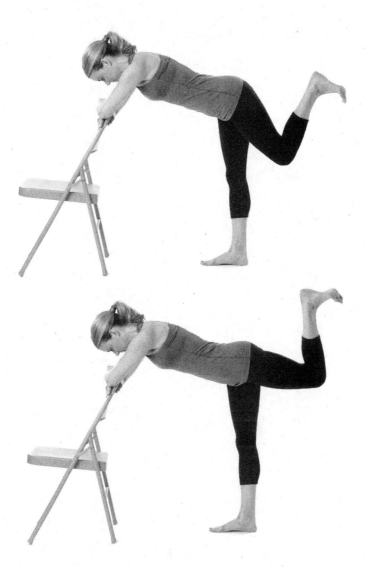

1. Start with both hands on the back of the chair and walk back until you can place your forearms on top, stacked on each other.

2. Keep your hips facing the floor and lift your left leg up behind you with the knee bent and heel facing the ceiling (your thigh should be parallel to the floor).

3. Pulse the left heel up an inch and back down an inch twenty times until you feel the burn in the back of the thigh.

4. Repeat on the right side, and perform 2 to 3 sets.

Dancer's Pose

Dancer's pose opens up the chest and shoulders as well as the fronts of the thighs. Dancer's pose feels so celebratory and makes me happy every time I do it. The pose is also great for building strength in the legs and core and for working on balance. The mudra we make with our hand by joining the thumb and forefinger celebrates the joining of the self with the larger community or universe.

Works Your: Legs, hips, abs, back, and arms

Try This: When you need a little cheering up; want to celebrate your life and accomplishments; feel stiff in the shoulders, back, or hip flexors; or need to work on your balance

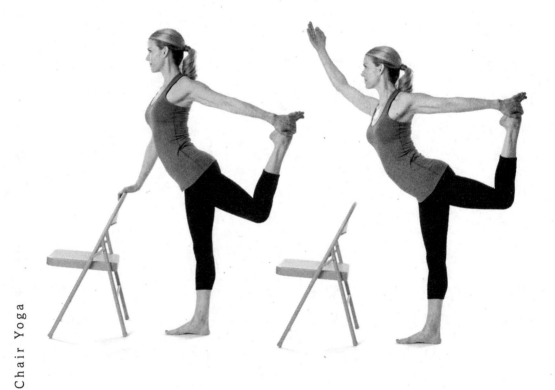

1. Start standing toward the left of the back of the chair. Place your right hand on the chairback and reach around with your left hand to catch the top of the left foot.

2. Bow the left leg behind you as you lean forward with the chest and open up the entire front body.

3. Once you feel steady, lift the right arm out in front of you and join the thumb and forefinger together.

4. Hold and breathe for 5 to 8 breaths. Repeat on the right side.

Shoulder and Triceps Stretch

One of the most common areas in which I see people storing stress (myself included) seems to be the shoulder and neck region. It's incredible how often I find myself with shoulders tensed up to my ears, like a second pair of earrings. Throughout the day try to catch yourself and remind yourself to relax the shoulders down again. This standing shoulder stretch is huge for releasing the arms, head, neck, and shoulder girdle.

Works Your: Upper back, shoulders, and arms

Try This: When you need a good release in the shoulders, feel a ton of pressure in your life and want a break, have been carrying heavy bags and have a moment to relax (possibly at the airport), or want some quiet time to yourself

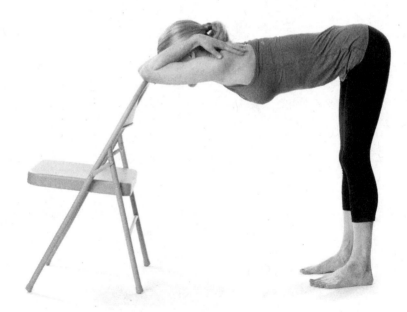

1. Start by standing facing the back of your chair.

2. Walk back far enough to place the back of the elbow region on the top of the chairback. Your upper body should be parallel to the floor.

3. Rest your hands on your shoulder blades and release into the hammock of the stretch. Make sure to keep your abs engaged and don't overarch the upper or lower back. You should feel the stretch primarily in the shoulders, upper back, and triceps.

4. Hold for 5 to 8 breaths.

Variation:

1. For an even deeper stretch, kneel on the floor facing the seat of your chair. Place a pillow under your knees if you need extra support.

2. Sit back a ways and rest the backs of the elbows on top of the seat.

3. Let the upper body release into the stretch while keeping the abdominals engaged.

4. Hold for 5 to 8 breaths.

Chaturanga Push-ups

Many beginner students have a challenging time performing chaturanga *correctly and not letting their shoulders round forward or their hips drop too low or lift too high in the pose. Practicing this narrow arm push-up with a chair is a great way to start to build strength while still maintaining good form.*

Works Your: Arms (especially the triceps), chest, and abs
Try This: When you want to get some quick energy

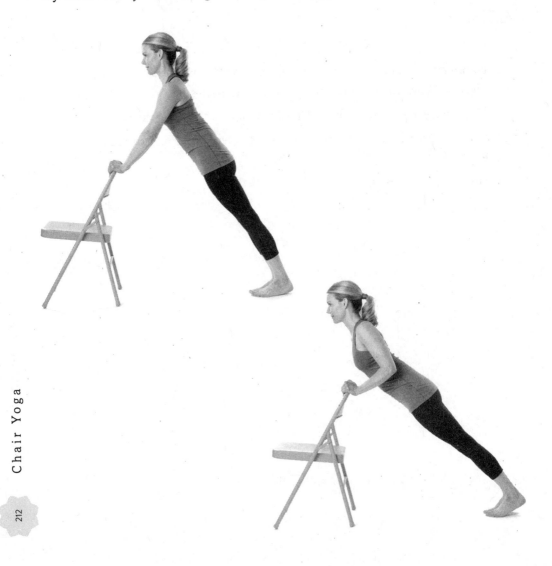

1. Start by standing at the back of your chair and place your hands on the chairback (make sure the chair is secure or locked in place).

2. Have your hands about shoulder-width apart and walk your feet back about two feet, forming an angle to the chair.

3. Inhale and lower your body toward the chair as you narrow your elbows behind you. Exhale and push back up to starting position.

4. Repeat for a set of 12 to 15 push-ups, and go for 2 to 3 sets if you have the time and stamina.

Variation:

1. As you build up strength in the upper body, try to do the push-ups using the seat of the chair so your body is closer to the floor and almost parallel.

2. Start with your hands on the seat (again make sure the chair is stable).

3. With hands shoulder-width apart, lower your chest toward the chair on an inhalation, narrowing the arms behind you and squeezing an imaginary grapefruit between the shoulder blades.

4. Exhale and press back up to the start of the push-up position. Repeat 12 to 15 times, and build up to 2 to 3 sets.

When I started practicing yoga, I discovered just how much stronger and toned I became, especially in the upper body. My mom was shocked when she first saw me supporting myself on my arms.

Chaturanga, the Sanskrit name for a yogi push-up, is one of the main postures that I credit for my upper body strength and tone.

Extended Side Angle

It's always so refreshing to stretch the side of your body and create space for the lungs to expand. Standing in extended side angle gives us the ability to really go deep into the side stretch and use our legs for support. I love doing it with a chair so I can balance myself and crank my torso around.

Works Your: Hips, thighs, buttocks, arms, abs, and shoulders
Try This: When you need some fresh air in the lungs, want to open up the torso and lengthen the waist, have energy to spare and want a good leg workout, or feel the need to expand in all directions.

1. Start in standing warrior II pose on your right side in front of the chair.
2. Place your right hand on the seat of the chair behind the right knee as you extend your left arm up overhead at a 45-degree angle and lean to your right.
3. Try to keep both sides of the waist long and the tops of the shoulders soft.
4. Feel the length and reach from the outer edge of the left foot all the way through to the left fingers. Hold for 5 to 8 breaths before coming up to stand and repeating on the other side.

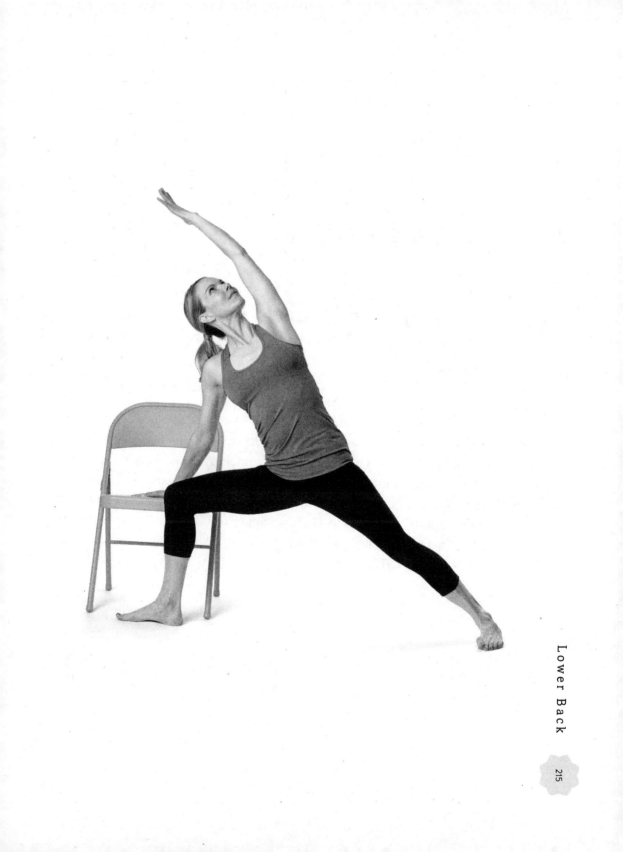

10

Putting It All Together

This chapter is designed to show you how you can combine the poses to get different results. The mix is endless and you can always experiment with building your own flows. Here are some of my favorite routines. Whether you're dealing with stress or digestive issues, looking to lose weight or unwind, these routines will help you to look and feel your best. Feel free to perform these routines whenever you want to. Keep track of your daily progress and notice how your mind and body start to change for the better.

Five-Minute Routines

There are so many moments in our day when we can find the time to sneak in some standing yoga postures. If you're on a phone call, why not hold a tree pose? While you're organizing your papers or reviewing a document or reading a letter, take turns holding the papers in opposite hands while doing a standing quadriceps stretch or dancer's pose. Lunges, warriors, and triangles can all be done using the chair for assistance while standing. You may even want to incorporate these poses into a pre- or post-workout using a park bench if you're going for a jog or walk in the park.

Five Minutes to De-stress • Five-Minute Sitting Abs
Five-Minute Face-lift • Five Minutes to Better Digestion
Five Minutes to More Energy • Five Minutes to Boost Your Immunity

Five Minutes to De-stress

This routine will help you relieve anxiety. You can do this whenever you need to de-stress or feel like you just can't focus. The breathing helps to center you. The cat/cow movement is rhythmic and rocking and calming for the nervous system. All the postures relieve stress in the shoulders and neck region. And taking a moment for a deep forward bend and some final relaxation quiets the mind.

1. Alternate nostril breathing (page 14)
2. Cat/cow (pages 26, 165)
3. High altar leans (page 80)
4. Clasped-hands head forward bow (page 51)
5. Backbend arch (page 164)
6. Roll downs (page 166)
7. Shoulder shrugs (page 70)
8. Head circles (page 46)
9. Final relaxation (page 250)

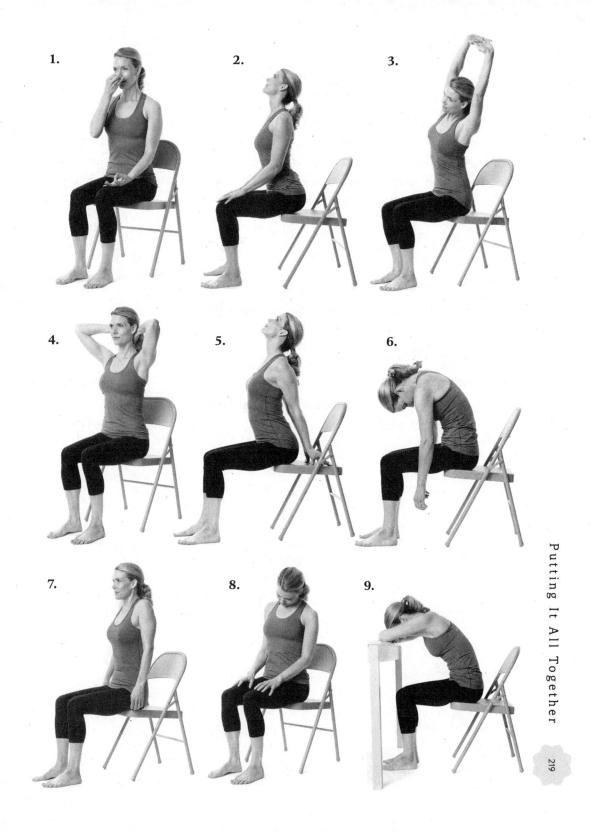

1.

2.

3.

4.

5.

6.

7.

8.

9.

Five-Minute Sitting Abs

Here's a great sequence to get your abs and core strong and in shape. You can do this whenever you want to tone and tighten your midsection or need some help supporting your lower back. All the abdominal moves work the core and transverse abdominals. The twist helps to tone the obliques, as do the side-to-sides. Straddle forward bend with twist also works the core deeply while also targeting the inner thighs.

1. Leg lifts (page 108)
2. Seat lifts (page 106)
3. Leg reaches and leg reaches with twists (page 110)
4. Bicycles (page 112)
5. Single leg stretch (page 114)
6. Scissors (page 116)
7. Side-to-side crunches with hands behind the head (page 124)
8. Straddle forward bend with twist (page 128)

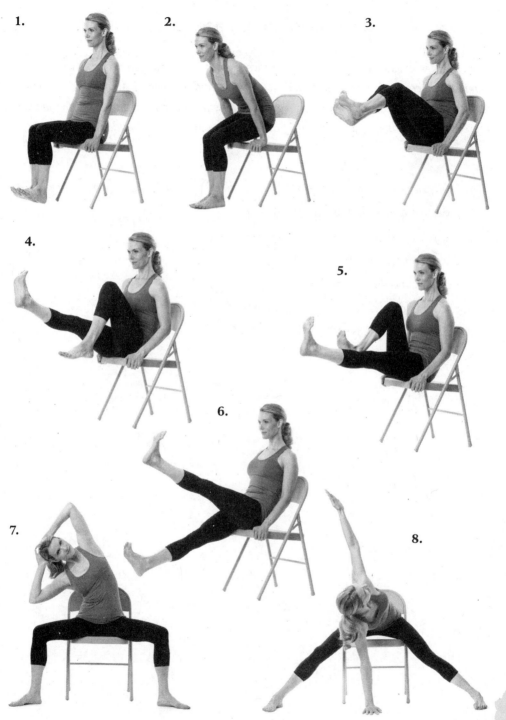

1.　2.　3.

4.　5.

6.

7.　8.

Five-Minute Face-Lift

Stretch and strengthen the muscles of your face to keep your facial features taut and younger looking. You can do a five-minute face-lift any time and anywhere! All of these movements with our eyes, mouth, and jaw help the muscles stay flexible and strong. Brushing the neck is great for eliminating the downward flow of gravity that we all dread.

1. Up/downs with eyes (page 54)
2. Side-to-sides with eyes (page 55)
3. Head back downward gaze (page 59)
4. Fishy face (page 60)
5. Lower jaw over top teeth (page 62)
6. Side-to-sides with lower jaw (page 63)
7. Wide smiles (page 65)
8. Neck brushing (page 50)

1.

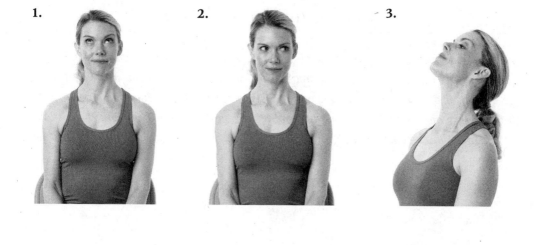

2.

3.

4.

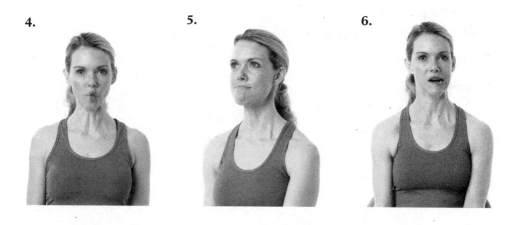

5.

6.

7.

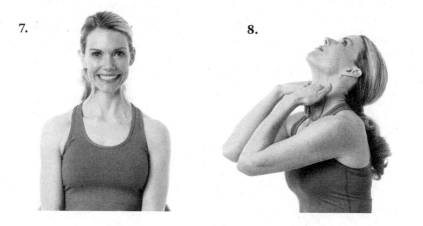

8.

Five Minutes to Better Digestion

Want to keep your digestive system running smoothly? Try this routine whenever you're feeling sluggish or backed up. Bhastrika breath is like stoking a fire. Circular movements help get things going down below. Moving our legs is another way to get digestion moving. Side bends stretch and twists squeeze our internal organs, both of which help with elimination. Standing up and lengthening the front body can clear things up as well and stimulate the digestive tract.

1. Bhastrika (page 17)
2. Pelvic tilts/circles (page 24)
3. Marching flow (page 38)
4. Extended side angle (page 214)
5. Chair twist (page 100)
6. Quad stretch (page 174)
7. Low lunge (page 180)
8. Warrior II (page 148)

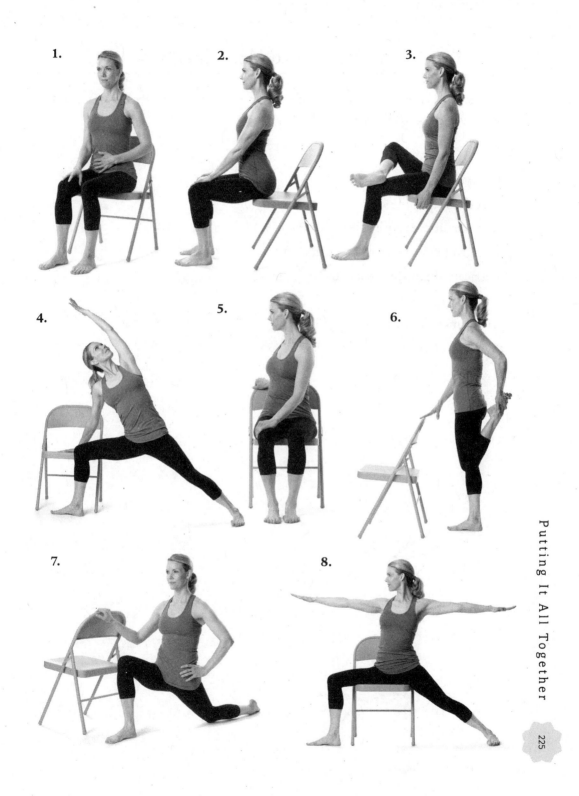

1.

2.

3.

4.

5.

6.

7.

8.

Five Minutes to More Energy

Here's an awesome quick routine to get you energized in no time. I personally love to do this around four o'clock when I need to reboot my system.

1. Kapalbhati (page 10)
2. Toe taps (page 135)
3. Sun salutation with side bends (page 36)
4. High altar triceps presses (page 78)
5. Triceps dips using seat of chair (page 82)
6. Tree (page 196)
7. Downward-facing dog (page 188)
8. Warrior III (150)

1.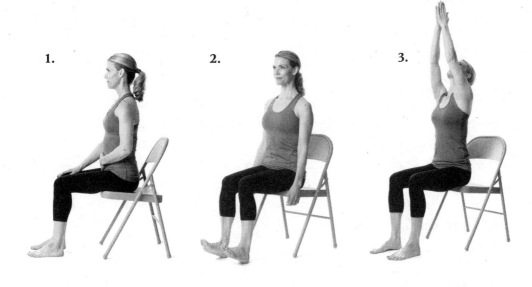

2.

3.

4.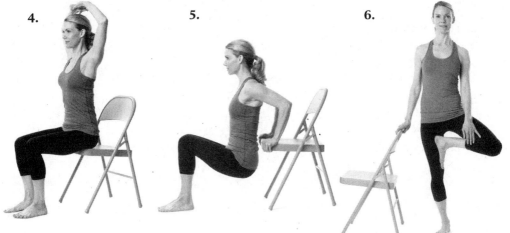

5.

6.

7.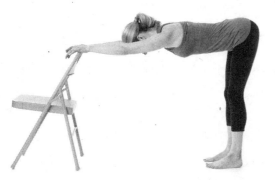

8.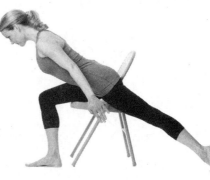

Five Minutes to Boost Your Immunity

When you're feeling a little run-down you can try this routine to stimulate the lymphatic system and boost your immunity. Ujjayi breathing is a wonderful way to get the blood flowing and oxygenate the lungs. Stretching out the neck and performing self-care remind you to take it easy on yourself and alleviate stress. Stress wreaks havoc on our immune system. Opening up the front body and arms keeps the chest open and our lungs clear. Lunge and warrior I clear the front body, and doing poses that work the larger muscle groups get our lymph and metabolic systems moving.

1. Ujjayi (page 8)
2. Held assisted stretches for side and angle (page 48)
3. Triceps stretch (page 86)
4. Cow face arms (page 74)
5. Lunge (page 152)
6. Warrior I (page 146)
7. Behind-the-back prayer hands (page 92)
8. Leg on ledge fold (page 158)

1.

2.

3.

4.

5.

6.

7.

8.

Ten-Minute Routines

Now that you're getting the hang of just how easy it is to sneak yoga in to your daily seated life, you'll love the renewed energy and focus you have. Once you're comfortable practicing for five minutes, try increasing the length to ten minutes. These ten-minute routines are easy to perform anywhere and any time of the day. You may even get some colleagues to join in on the fun with you. I often do some chair yoga routines when my son is playing on the floor. He gets such a kick out of it and will try mimicking me in the poses. Yoga is beneficial for everyone of all ages and at every stage of your life. I found the seated ten-minute chair workouts to be just what the doctor ordered during my third trimester pregnant with twins. I really didn't have much stamina or strength once I was in my final stages of a pregnancy with multiples, and yet I craved my yoga practice. Chair yoga was the perfect solution for me. I love these ten-minute routines and often find myself adding on even more time. Give these a try and of course once you're a chair yogi, have fun and come up with your own routines combining any of the exercises in this book.

Ten Minutes to More Energy • Ten Minutes to Less Stress
Ten Minutes to Unwind • Ten Minutes to Ease Back Pain
Ten Minutes to Happiness • Ten Minutes to Weight Loss

Ten Minutes to More Energy

On days when you have more time or in the morning when you're starting your day out, here is an energizing routine you can perform. You start out warming up the legs and then move into sun salutations. Ankle to knee, goddess, and warrior II poses open up the hips and work the larger muscles. Triceps dips strengthen the arms and get the heart rate up. Side leans open the lungs to get more oxygen in them. Downward dog brings blood flow to the brain, and triangle and tree are two great standing postures for energy and focus.

1. Dancing cat (page 28)
2. Sun salutation arms (page 30)
3. Sun salutation with folds (page 32)
4. Ankle to knee (page 140)
5. Goddess squat (page 154)
6. Warrior II (page 148)
7. Triceps dips using seat of chair (page 82)
8. Side leans with wrist pull (page 81)
9. Downward-facing dog (page 188)
10. Pigeon on chair (page 186)
11. Triangle (page 198)
12. Tree (page 196)

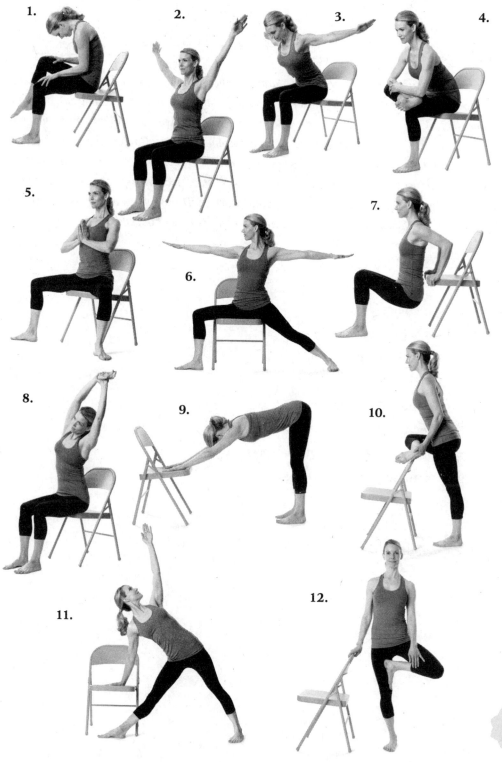

1. 2. 3. 4.

5. 6. 7.

8. 9. 10.

11. 12.

Stress is inevitable and we encounter it daily. It's how we manage our stress that matters. Yoga is instrumental in managing stress, and doing this ten-minute routine daily or a few times a week can help you calm down and relieve stress and tension. Viloma breathing immediately kicks the parasympathetic nervous system into gear. Circling the eyes gives our brain something to focus on and relieves eye tension. The other exercises release pent-up energy in our legs and feet, tension in our neck and shoulders. Working out our body with challenging exercises such as chaturanga and warrior III pose gives us a sense of accomplishment, which helps us feel more in control in other areas of our life.

1.   Viloma (page 19)
2.   Eye circles (page 56)
3.   Foot circles (page 133)
4.   Head circles (page 46)
5.   Hand pulls (page 90)
6.   Shoulder shrugs (page 70)
7.   Shoulder stretch (arm across front) (page 71)
8.   Eagle arms (with variations) (page 72)
9.   Chaturanga push-ups (page 212)
10. Warrior III (page 150)
11. Forward hang (page 190)
12. Standing side stretch (page 192)

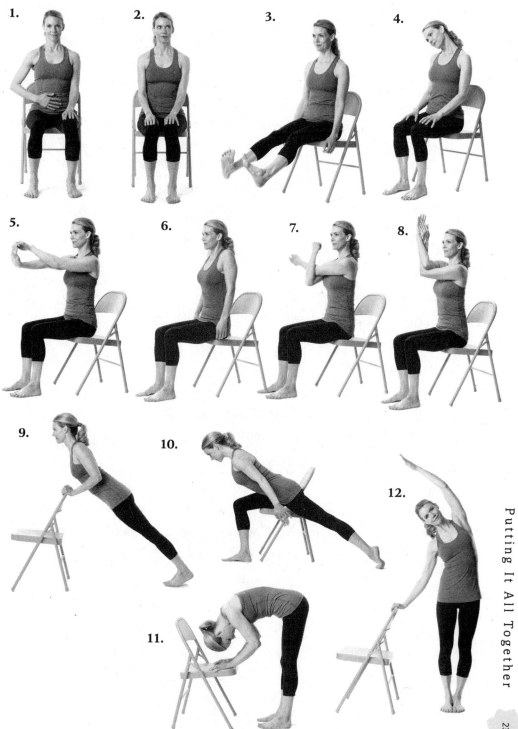

1. 2. 3. 4.

5. 6. 7. 8.

9. 10.

11. 12.

On days when you just want a gentle practice to help you unwind, the chair is the perfect prop. Take your time with each pose and close the eyes when it feels good. Releasing the neck and feet are both very soothing. Letting tension out of the hands and wrists is extremely therapeutic. Quiet forward bends relax the mind and remind us to slow down. Putting our legs up and letting the blood flow in reverse feels pretty amazing too. Gentle twists and side bends help us to unwind and release tension in the body.

1. Cat/cow (pages 26, 165)
2. Backbend arch (page 164)
3. Side-to-sides with waist (page 118)
4. Clasped-hands head forward bow (page 51)
5. Squeeze/spread (page 137)
6. Point/flex (page 134)
7. 1-2-3-4 wrist workout (page 85)
8. Goddess side stretch and twist (page 122)
9. Straddle forward bend (page 126)
10. Lower jaw over top teeth (page 62)
11. Sithali (page 21)
12. Shoulder and triceps stretch (kneeling variation) (page 210)
13. Final relaxation (can be head on desk or you can choose to do back relief pose [page 170] with your legs on the chair) (page 250)

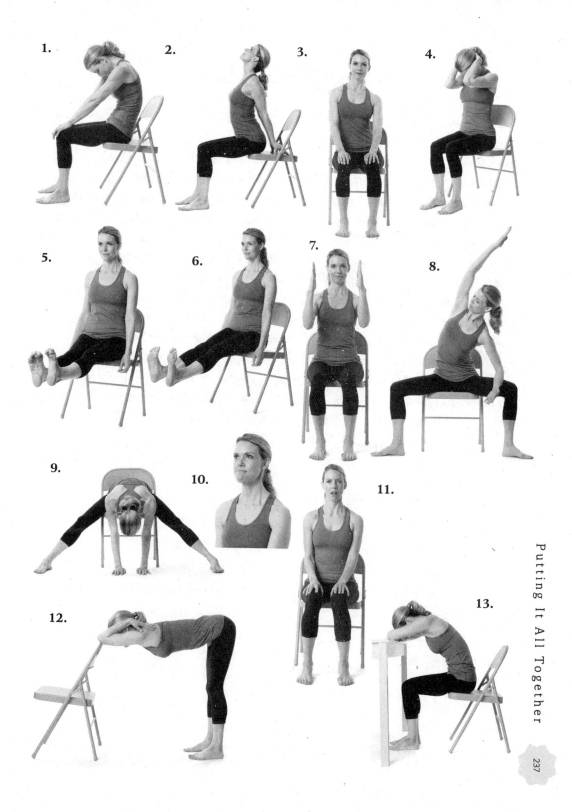

1.

2.

3.

4.

5.

6.

7.

8.

9.

10.

11.

12.

13.

237

Back pain can be debilitating, and it's always wise to consult with your doctor if you've been suffering for a while and find it difficult to do normal activities. Yoga is one tool that can help ease back pain, strengthen the core, and lengthen the spine while also stretching tight muscles that can pull on the back. If your doctor gives you the green light to keep moving, these chair exercises are ideal for you. Start slowly and always listen to your breath. If you feel pain, stop and breathe. If there is mild discomfort, that is natural and you can move your way through it. Over time your back will thank you for all the TLC you give it. Sitting for prolonged periods of time isn't great for our back or posture, so make sure you include some of these movements in your daily seated life as often as you can.

All of these movements warm up the spine and open up the body. Pelvic tilts/circles, side-to-sides, leg lifts, and butt squeezes all strengthen the abs and pelvic floor muscles and loosen up the back. Tight hips can do a number on the back, and cow legs pose is great for stretching the hips and external rotators. Twists and side bends are also awesome for stretching the spine, but be gentle on the twists if you feel it's too much for your back. Tight hip flexors pull on the lower back and upper back; lunging opens up the hip flexors and fronts of thighs. Backbend strengthens and supports the lower back; and letting the legs rest on the chair takes pressure off the back.

1. Pelvic tilts/circles (page 24)
2. Side-to-sides with waist (page 118)
3. Straight back fold (page 156)
4. Advanced hamstring stretch (page 160)
5. Leg lifts (page 108)
6. Butt squeezes (page 145)
7. Cow legs (page 144)
8. Behind-the-back prayer hands (page 92)
9. Side bends (page 103)
10. Standing twist (page 194)
11. Lunge (page 176)
12. Backbend (page 171)
13. Back relief (page 170)

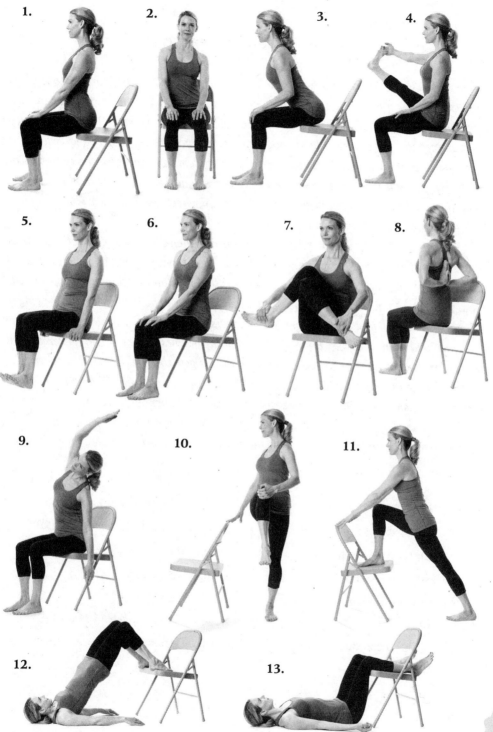

1.

2.

3.

4.

5.

6.

7.

8.

9.

10.

11.

12.

13.

Ten Minutes to Happiness

Yoga makes me so happy, and yoga can make you happy! I rarely hear someone say he wishes he hadn't gone to yoga class and opened up and stretched his body and connected with his breath. Even my biggest yoga skeptics will thank me and say, "Wow, I really need to be doing more of that," or "I felt so good after taking your class." Yoga releases feel-good endorphins in the body and relaxes our nervous system, and the breath oxygenates our body. Breathing is the best drug in town and it's free and healthy! This routine will boost your spirit any time you want to get happy or feel happier. Chances are you will inspire your office mates to start joining in too.

You start off by freeing up tension in the eyes and then do wide smiles with the mouth. Just the act of pretending to smile makes us happy. Lion's roar may not be doable if you're in public, but letting out a mighty roar and getting rid of stale air and things holding you back is so freeing and fun. Working our feet and brain forces us to be in the moment. Tracing the alphabet with each foot is challenging, which rewards our pleasure centers as adults when we learn and do new things. Flipped clasped hands is another one of those exercises that kind of messes with the brain, and everyone always gets a smile out of it. Backbends are known antidepressants and circling in goddess stimulates creativity. Tight hamstrings are always a downer, so opening them up and stretching the lower body brings us joy. Standing twists help us see all perspectives and change our point of view when we might be feeling down. And ending with dancer's pose is the best way to celebrate our life and feel happy.

1. Diagonals (page 58)
2. Wide smiles (page 65)
3. Lion's roar (page 66)
4. Alphabet (page 138)
5. Sun Salutation with twists (page 34)
6. Flipped clasped hands (page 88)
7. Backbend arch (page 164)
8. Goddess circles (page 120)
9. Scale pose (page 107)
10. Downward dog arms (page 96)
11. Standing twist (page 194)
12. Dancer's pose (page 209)

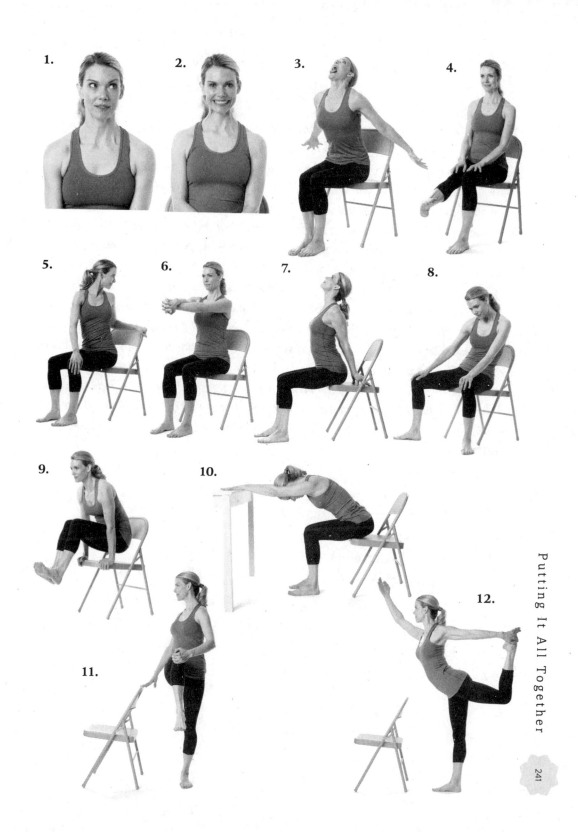

1. 2. 3. 4.

5. 6. 7. 8.

9. 10.

11. 12.

Ten Minutes to Weight Loss

Yoga is all about mindfulness and connecting with the body. When people start a yoga practice, there is often a huge change in how they feed their body. Yoga will help you make better choices about what you eat and how it affects your body, mood, energy, and physicality. The postures in yoga work our muscles in new ways, and you boost your metabolism when you have to hold postures and develop new strength. Flexibility and mobility allow us to move more freely and do more in our life, which naturally sets us up for more activity. Start incorporating this weight-loss routine into your life and notice the subtle changes that take place in your body. Yoga isn't a quick fix, though; it's a lifelong practice that over time truly helps you to cherish your body and become the best you can be.

You start out stoking the metabolism with kapalbhati breathing before moving into some warm-up flows that get the heart rate up and the blood flowing. Ankle to knee opens up the hips and large muscle groups. Next you move on to abdominal work and then the inner thighs. Side leans whittle the waist and warrior II is a stellar pose for working the entire body. Chaturanga is the best way to tone the arms and abs and burn some major calories. Butt lifts and figure 4 work the glutes and boost the buttocks. You cool off with a standing forward bend stretch for each leg and finish by stretching out the sides again to keep the body energized.

1. Kapalbhati (page 10)
2. Dancing cat (page 28)
3. Marching flow (page 38)
4. Ankle to knee (page 140)
5. Bicycles (page 112)
6. Leg reaches and leg reaches with twist (page 110)
7. High altar leans (page 80)
8. Warrior II (page 148)
9. Chaturanga push-ups (page 212)
10. Butt lifts (page 206)
11. Figure 4 (page 175)
12. Intense side stretch (page 184)

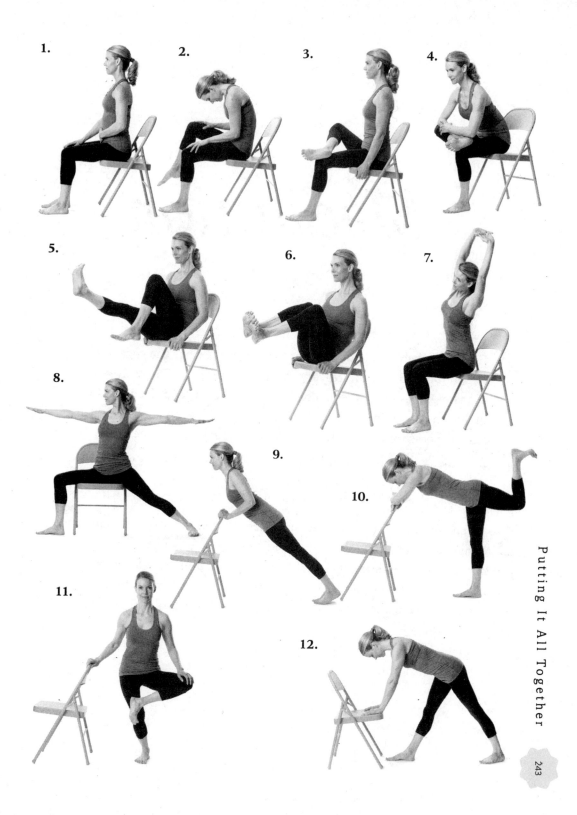

1.

2.

3.

4.

5.

6.

7.

8.

9.

10.

11.

12.

243

11

Meditation

Creating a daily meditation routine can be life altering. The yoga postures I've introduced you to are very meditative in and of themselves. Yoga asana prepares us for meditation by setting the stage for focusing on the breath and preparing the body to sit erect and with good posture. And just like the poses throughout the book, you can meditate anywhere.

So often throughout our day we are disconnected from the present moment. When you start moving the body mindfully while fully focusing on the breath, you will find how centering it is and your body and mind will feel more peaceful and at ease. The yoga postures also help release the body of excess tension, so when you sit you can have more freedom and won't be bothered by aches in the physical body.

Meditation is mostly about giving your mind a rest from all of its millions of thoughts. You may have heard the term "monkey mind." Meditation teaches us to slow the monkey down for a few seconds so we can get clearer on what we want and need in our lives. The monkey just needs to take a break on a branch every now and then and do nothing, instead of swinging from vine to vine and jumping up and down.

"So how do I meditate?" you might ask. Really all you need to do is carve out some time each day, whether it's one minute, five minutes, or twenty minutes, to sit and observe the breath. Our breath is our greatest tool for changing our mind state, and it's at our ready whenever we need it. The chair is a perfect place to meditate if you use the proper seat: feet flat on the floor hip-width apart, sitz bones anchored, shoulders down and back, and spine nice and tall. (If we slouch, our breath is diminished.)

Once you find a nice, tall, comfortable seat, you can close your eyes and rest your hands on your lap. I like to turn my palms up and join the thumb and forefinger. When our palms are open we are receptive, and it also helps flip the lungs open. The mudra of thumb and forefinger is just a nice gesture to remind us that we are stopping to do something important and more formal than just sitting. Once you are set, start to observe the breath.

Watch the inhalation and the exhalation. That's it! Just watch each breath. Repeat in your mind, "Breathing in, I am breathing in. Breathing out, I am breathing out." When the mind begins to wander, rein it back in and repeat the phrase again. You can also simplify it to "breath in, breath out," "breathe in, breathe out," or the Sanskrit *soham,* which translates to "I am that."

It is totally natural and normal for the mind to go off on tangents. Just keep bringing it back. Set a timer and start with anywhere from one to five minutes. Keep adding time until you can eventually get up to fifteen or twenty minutes. You might find it easier to stick to a routine if you pick the same time every day, but it truly doesn't matter when or where you meditate. You might be feeling tired, stressed, pressured, or depressed—these are all great times to meditate. I feel the more I meditate, the more I want to. Start slowly and build up.

I've found myself meditating in the airport, when I was nursing my son, at the doctor's office, and in my bed. If you are at a desk all day long, you may want to pick the midday slump time to establish a practice. Four o'clock is a great time to rejuvenate the mind. You can meditate briefly before a meal if you get anxious around food. You can meditate before or after a yoga practice. You can meditate before a big presentation. Meditation is truly a way to just reset the mind and continue working on being present and open to every precious moment of your life.

Meditation has been shown to reduce blood pressure, lower the heart rate, calm the nervous system, enhance creativity, and help with stress. Meditation is helpful for coping with all life throws our way. It helps us build a stronger sense of self. When you are sitting in your seat wherever you are, you can always take a few moments to close your eyes and focus on your breath. No one else can breathe for you.

Besides just focusing on the inhalation and exhalation, here are a few other meditations you can do to help calm the mind and channel your energy.

Lake Meditation

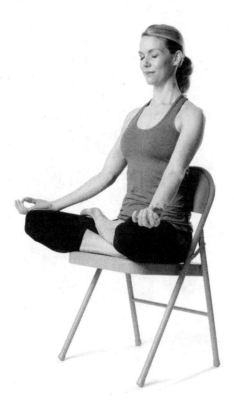

Sit still with your spine straight. Start to observe your breath. Imagine your mind is a mountain lake. Thoughts are like stones being thrown in the water, creating ripples and bringing sediment up from the bottom of the lake. Imagine placing the stones back on the bank and letting the ripples cease. Eventually the water becomes completely clear and so does the mind.

4-7-8 Breathing

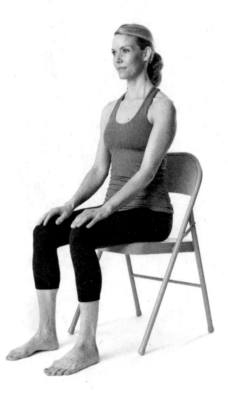

Sometimes for us type-A personalities it helps to focus on a count. This breathing technique helps us meditate by counting the beats of the breath. Sit up nice and tall with your hands resting on your lap. Inhale for a count of four, hold for a count of seven, and exhale for a count of eight. The exhalation being the longest helps to really clear everything out. We often hold on to residual stale air, and we cannot fully fill up with new, fresh air and thoughts unless we completely empty out.

Rainbow Meditation with Kapalbhati

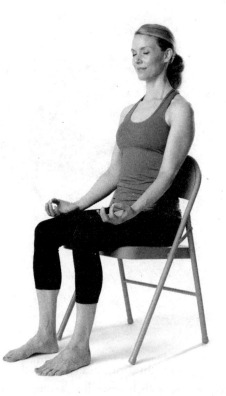

This is one of my favorite visualizations/meditations. Sit at the edge of your chair with your feet planted firmly. Lift your arms up so they create a giant V shape above your head. Press your fingers to your palms and open the thumbs out so they are pointing toward each other. Now imagine a giant rainbow arching from thumb to thumb.

Count out a round of one hundred rapid kapalbhati exhalations. After your last exhale, inhale a giant breath and hold it in for as long as you can. Keep inflating the chest and lifting it up to your chin as you bow your head forward. Once you can no longer hold the breath, touch your thumbs and pop a giant golden water balloon above you, and let the gifts rain down from above as your palms come back onto your lap, facing upward in a gesture of receptivity.

Final Relaxation

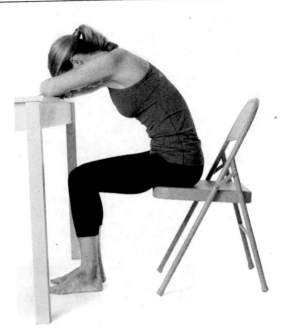

Final relaxation isn't quite meditation, but it can feel very meditative. Final relaxation is like a deep state of rest without falling asleep. You don't have to focus on the breath but just let it happen. We typically take final relaxation at the end of a class, but you can stop what you're doing any time of the day and give yourself a rest.

When I was very young, there was always time at school for milk and cookies and then a little nap. I think as adults we take only the work and assignment aspects from school and focus on them way too much. Wouldn't it be nice to have a time of day, every day, when you had a cup of tea with a nice handful of almonds, or a square of good dark chocolate, and then took a little rest?

If you're at your desk and feel comfortable doing so, fold your arms one on top of the other and place your forehead down on top of them. Close your eyes and listen to the oceanic sound of the breath. If you don't have a desk in front of you, just sit back in your chair without fully slumping but in a comfortable position. Your hands can rest gently on your knees and you can close your eyes and relax.

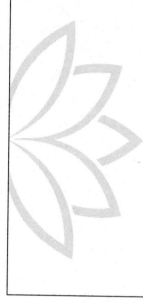

For more guided meditations, check out these websites and apps:

Websites

Meditate ON (yeahdave.com/meditate-on/)
Ziva Meditation (zivameditation.com)

Apps

Headspace
The Mindfulness App
Buddhify 2
Stop, Breathe & Think
Smiling Mind
Akasha

Acknowledgments

I't's hard to know where to begin when it comes to expressing my sincere gratitude for everyone who has supported me on my journey. A wide-eyed girl from Pocatello, Idaho, ends up in the Big Apple to attend acting school at New York University and soon discovers this incredible thing called yoga. I can't go without thanking the very first people who introduced me to the yoga practice, Nikki Costello, Sharon Gannon and David Life, Cyndi Lee, Richard Freeman, Dana Flynn, Baron Baptiste, and Peter Rizzo to name a few. Or those who continue to inspire me on my path as I constantly learn and hone my practice and teaching as much as I can, Kelly Kane, Lisa Landphair, Nevine Michaan, David Romanelli, Lori Head, and Carey Macaleer to name a few more. My profession and art is a constant study of the body and mind connection and I love to soak in as much knowledge and firsthand experience as I can.

I also need to thank my faithful clients, from Steve Martin to Anne Ford, Wendy Breck and Lee Auchincloss, to Christine Stiller, Savannah Guthrie, Emily DiDonato, Emilia Clarke and LeAnn Rimes, Craig Balsam, Craig McDean, Sean Fahey, Pip Coburn, and all of my Crunch, Equinox, Clay, and Reebok students who have remained loyal and who all have such great fun while I put them into precarious positions or try out new exercises on them. Many of them have opened doors for me, like Tina Fey, who helped cast me in a guest spot on *30 Rock,* to Sam Hoffman, who recently had me play a small part in his film *Humor Me.* So many students of mine have promoted me or led me to incredible opportunities and I can't thank them enough.

I have sincere respect and gratitude for other writers and I thank my family at *Health* magazine and Clare McHugh for helping me hone my skills over the years as a writer. I'm also grateful to Rita Treiger, who gave me one of my first editorial jobs at *Fit Yoga,* as well as Amanda Altman, who continues to have me contribute to *Pilates Style* magazine. I'm thankful to Scott Mebus and Maggie Nemser for believing in my work as we filmed four DVDs for MTV, which soon launched my career as a spokeswoman, DVD star, and host. I'm thankful to my first business partners, Matt Yu and Tony Aufiero, who helped me understand the business side of being a yogi and helped me produce my very own collection of DVDs. I'm grateful for my amazing web gals Ophira Edut and Liz Theresa for their help with my website over the years. I'm happy for my collaborators who have great ideas and help to make things happen like Daphne Borowski and her team, who produced my app and helped me with photo shoots and DVD production as well. I'm thankful for angels who come in and out of my life like Clay Enos, who always helped me with anything I needed—from photography to travel and life lessons.

I'm thankful to Cara Bedick for approaching me with this amazing idea and the team at HarperCollins including Diahann Sturge in design, Emily Homonoff in publicity, and Molly Waxman in marketing. I'm thankful to Sue Hitzmann for all of her support. I'm thrilled with Chris Fanning's work on the photos for the book and grateful for Ann Pennington for her styling, makeup, and hair for the shoot. She always helps me look great! I am also thankful to Alison Graham, Sharon House, and their team at AJGpr for all of their help with marketing.

I'm grateful to all of my friends who have understood the times I've been too busy to go out partying because I'm at home writing or sleeping since I have to get up at 5 a.m. to teach the next day. I'm grateful for all of my childhood friends who to this day still acknowledge me and support me from near or afar to my grown adult friends and mommy friends who help me relax a little and stop to smell the roses and play with the kiddos. I'm grateful for my husband, who's never held me back from traveling off to teach or shoot yoga videos or host on the Home Shopping Network, who's had to shoot pictures for me for Instagram or film videos for my own site or YouTube channel and doesn't complain, someone who I actually met through a yoga student who set us up . . . once again I have yoga to thank for all of my circumstances in life!

Most important, I'm grateful beyond what words can express for my family. My mom and my dad have always believed in me and supported me in so many ways. My dad used to stay up with me into the wee hours of the night as I worked with my Virgo perfection on writing assignments in high school. My dad still to this day reads over whatever I've written and patiently helps me figure out the right wording for what I'm trying to say. My mom is my best friend and I couldn't do half of what I do without her. She flies all the way across the country to help out with my adorable son Timothy when needed so I can pursue my passion and career. She has never let me give up on my dreams. My brothers have been incredible to me and my older brother has pretty much been everything from my manager to my business coach to my best friend. My younger brother has always had my back and makes sure I stay grounded. My son has changed my life in ways beyond imaginable and I never thought it could be possible to love someone as much as I love him. Poor kid has heard the clacking of my keys as I type since he was a wee baby nursing on my breast while I tried to balance him on my lap just right so I could get my thoughts on paper.

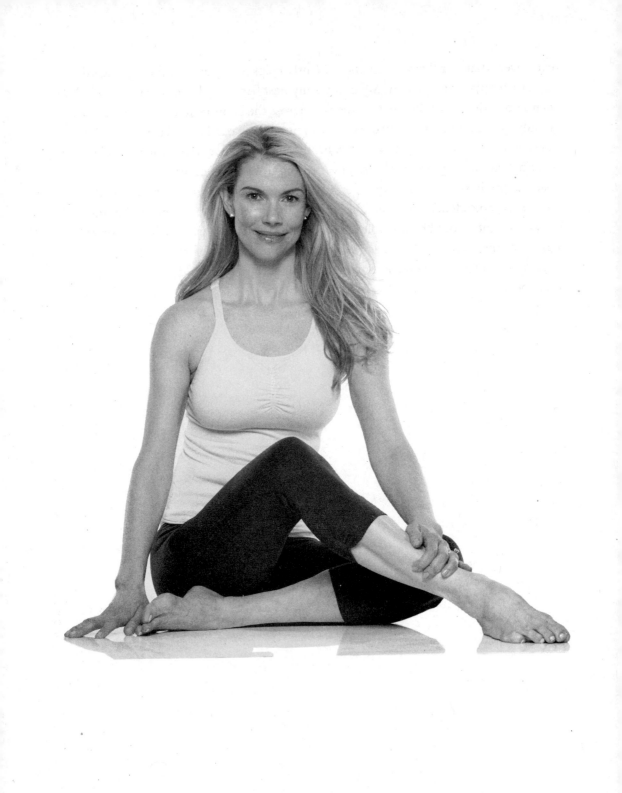

About the Author

KRISTIN McGEE discovered yoga back in the early 1990s when it was recommended to her as a way to connect with her body. After studying with some of the world's most renowned instructors, Kristin created her own style of yoga that was an instant hit for its upbeat, refreshingly hip approach.

Kristin is a yoga and Pilates teacher, celebrity trainer, and host and star of more than one hundred fitness DVDs, including MTV's *Yoga* and *Power Yoga*. Kristin has appeared on *Good Morning America,* Fox's *Good Day New York, The Tyra Banks Show,* and the *Today* show, as well as CNN's Headline News and HSN, as a fitness consultant, and she has been on the covers of *Pilates Style* and *Fit Yoga* magazines. Kristin is a contributing editor for *Health* magazine and has written for publications such as *Shape, Fitness, Self, InStyle, Women's Health, Body & Soul,* and *Prevention* and websites such as *Yahoo! Health* and *Huffington Post.* Her clients have included celebrities such as Steve Martin, Tina Fey, LeAnn Rimes, Ben and Christine Stiller, Bethenny Frankel, and Savannah Guthrie, just to name a few. Kristin is an avid spokesperson for companies and causes that promote health and wellness. She lives in New York.

Index

Index